TOXICOLOGY EMERGENCY: A PRACTICAL GUIDE TO DIAGNOSIS AND MANAGEMENT

Comprehensive Strategies for Managing Drug Overdoses, Environmental Exposures, and Envenomations

Walter C. Jeffords, MD, FAAEM, FACEP

Copyright © 2024 by Walter C. Jeffords, MD, FAAEM, FACEP

All rights reserved. No part of this book may be reproduced, stored in a retrieval system, or transmitted in any form or by any means, electronic, mechanical, photocopying, recording, or otherwise, without the prior written permission of the publisher, except as provided by U.S. copyright law. For permission requests, contact the publisher.

TOXICOLOGY EMERGENCY: A PRACTICAL GUIDE TO DIAGNOSIS AND MANAGEMENT
Comprehensive Strategies for Managing Drug Overdoses, Environmental Exposures, and Envenomations

Walter C. Jeffords, MD, FAAEM, FACEP
2024

Preface

Toxicology is a critical branch of medicine that encompasses a broad range of complex and potentially life-threatening conditions. As an emergency medicine specialist and clinical toxicologist, I have spent many years treating patients who present with a variety of toxicological emergencies, ranging from drug overdoses and environmental exposures to venomous bites and stings. Over the years, it has become increasingly clear that while toxicology emergencies are often urgent and challenging, a systematic, evidence-based approach to diagnosis and management can significantly improve patient outcomes.

Toxicoxicology Emergency: A Practical Guide to Diagnosis and Management was written with the goal of providing a comprehensive, user-friendly resource for clinicians on the front lines of managing toxicological emergencies.

This book is intended for emergency physicians, residents, toxicologists, paramedics, and other healthcare professionals who are tasked with diagnosing and managing patients with toxicological conditions. Whether you're a seasoned clinician or a trainee, this guide aims to be an essential companion in the assessment and management of these critical patients.

The primary focus of this book is on the most common and urgent toxicological conditions encountered in the emergency department, including drug overdoses, environmental exposures, and envenomations. It draws from the latest evidence-based practices, clinical trials, and my own years of clinical experience to provide practical strategies for the management of these cases.

The structure of this book is designed to allow readers to quickly access relevant, concise, and actionable information. The chapters are organized into clear sections that focus on individual topics, providing detailed guidance on recognizing signs and symptoms, conducting diagnostic evaluations, and implementing the most effective treatments. In addition, we delve into advanced strategies such as the use of antidotes, extracorporeal therapies, and the role of supportive care.

In addressing drug overdoses, we explore both common and less typical substances, offering detailed information on the pharmacokinetics, toxicity profiles, and clinical management of the most frequently encountered agents. Environmental exposures—ranging from toxic chemicals to pollutants and industrial hazards—are examined, with practical approaches for assessing risk and treatment. Envenomations, whether from snakes, insects, or marine organisms, also receive in-depth coverage, with expert guidance on species identification, clinical evaluation, and therapeutic interventions.

One of the key objectives of this book is to present complex toxicological issues in an easily understandable and clinically relevant manner. While the field of toxicology is often seen as complex and esoteric, I have aimed to simplify concepts without sacrificing scientific rigor. The practical approach taken here allows readers to quickly understand the key principles and apply them to real-world clinical situations.

Throughout the text, I emphasize a holistic approach to patient care, addressing not just the physiological effects of toxins but also the psychological and social aspects of toxicology emergencies. Many patients suffering from toxicological exposures or overdoses present with additional complexities, including substance use disorders, mental health issues, or underlying chronic conditions. A comprehensive understanding of these factors is essential for providing effective care, and this book strives to prepare clinicians to address them in a sensitive and thorough manner.

Additionally, this book reflects the latest advancements in the field of toxicology, including novel antidotes, therapeutic agents, and cutting-edge diagnostic tools. As new treatments and protocols emerge, it is essential that clinicians stay up-to-date, and I have included the most current information to ensure that this guide remains a relevant resource in clinical practice.

This work is the culmination of years of clinical experience, scholarly research, and collaboration with colleagues in emergency medicine and toxicology. I am grateful to the many professionals who have shared their insights and expertise, which have contributed to the richness of this text.

Finally, I want to acknowledge the significant role of emergency care teams in the management of toxicological emergencies. Whether it's the emergency physician, toxicologist, nurse, or paramedic, the multidisciplinary approach to care is what makes successful patient outcomes possible. It is my hope that this book serves as a valuable tool in helping all members of the healthcare team deliver the highest level of care to patients experiencing toxicological emergencies.

Walter C. Jeffords, MD, FAAEM, FACEP
Clinical Toxicologist and Emergency Medicine Specialist
2024

Preface
Table of content
List of Abbreviations

Table of Contents

Chapter 1: Comprehensive Approach to the Poisoned Patient

1. Introduction to Poisoning Emergencies
Understanding the Spectrum of Toxicological Emergencies
Significance of Early Recognition

2. Key Considerations in Poison Management
Self-Poisoning as a Reflection of Underlying Issues
Diverse Clinical Presentations of Toxicity
Risk Assessment as a Predictor of Clinical Outcomes

3. Principles of Supportive Care
Importance of Stabilization and Monitoring

Organ-Specific Support Strategies

4. Gastrointestinal Decontamination
Risk-Benefit Analysis in Decontamination
Role of Activated Charcoal and Other Techniques
Delayed Interventions in Select Cases

5. Management of Toxicology Cases
Essential Techniques and Interventions
Antidote Use: Indications and Limitations
Evidence-Based Practices in Toxicology

6. Conclusion and Key Takeaways
Summary of Best Practices
Importance of a Multidisciplinary Approach

Chapter 2: Cardiovascular Drug Toxicity Management

1. Introduction to Cardiovascular Drug Toxicity
Overview of High-Risk Cardiovascular Agents
Common Clinical Presentations

2. Life-Threatening Risks in Overdoses
Calcium Channel Blockers (CCBs)
β-Blockers
Sodium Channel Blockers
Digoxin

3. Management Strategies for CCB and
β-Blocker Toxicity
Aggressive Circulatory Support
Role of Hyperinsulinemic Euglycemic Therapy

4. Delayed Onset in Slow-Release Formulations
Recognizing and Managing Slow-Release CCB Toxicity
Timing and Monitoring Considerations

5. Gastrointestinal Decontamination
Whole-Bowel Irrigation for Slow-Release CCB Overdoses
Early Decontamination Techniques

6. Sodium Channel Blocker Overdose Management

Sodium Bicarbonate Therapy
Hyperventilation as a Therapeutic Strategy

7. Digoxin Toxicity and its Treatment
Early Recognition and Intervention
Use of Digoxin-Specific Antibody Fab Fragments

8. Supportive Management in Clonidine Poisoning
Key Principles of Supportive Care
Addressing Symptoms and Vital Organ Support

9. Intravenous Lipid Emulsion (ILE) Therapy
Indications for ILE in Local Anesthetic Toxicity
Limitations in Broader Drug Overdose Applications

10. Conclusion and Key Takeaways
Summary of Evidence-Based Practices
Emphasis on Early Intervention and Multidisciplinary Care

Chapter 3: Antipsychotic Drugs

1. Introduction
Therapeutic Use and Patient Adherence Challenges

2. Adverse Effects of Antipsychotics
Common Side Effects at Therapeutic Doses
Extrapyramidal Symptoms (EPS) and Drug Class Differences

3. High-Risk Antipsychotics
Clozapine: Agranulocytosis and Myocarditis
Monitoring Protocols for Safe Usage

4. Toxicity and Overdose
Central Nervous System (CNS) Depression
Cardiovascular Complications in Overdose

5. Cardiac Concerns
Amisulpride and QT Interval Prolongation
Risk of Torsades de Pointes

6. Management Strategies
Supportive Care for Antipsychotic Overdose

Evidence-Based Interventions

7. Neuroleptic Malignant Syndrome (NMS)
Clinical Presentation and Diagnosis
Critical Timelines for Effective Treatment

Chapter 4: Antidepressant Drugs

1. Introduction
Overview of Antidepressant Toxicity

2. Tricyclic Antidepressants (TCAs)
Cardiovascular Toxicity and Seizures
Sodium Bicarbonate Therapy

3. Selective Serotonin Reuptake Inhibitors (SSRIs)
Overdose Symptoms and Serotonin Toxicity
QT Prolongation and Torsades de Pointes Risks

4. Selective Noradrenaline Reuptake Inhibitors
Serotonin and Sympathomimetic Toxicity
Delayed Cardiovascular Effects

5. Monoamine Oxidase Inhibitors (MAOIs)
Delayed Sympathomimetic Stimulation
Intensive Care Requirements

Chapter 5: Lithium

1. Chronic Lithium Toxicity
Diagnosis and Neurological Manifestations
Role of Renal Impairment

2. Acute Lithium Overdose
Symptoms and Management
Prognosis Based on Dosage

3. Acute-on-Chronic Toxicity
Risks of Neurotoxicity and Monitoring

4. Hemodialysis for Lithium Elimination
Indications and Protocols

Chapter 6: Paracetamol Poisoning

1. Epidemiology and Prevalence

2. Risk Assessment Using the Paracetamol Treatment Nomogram

3. N-Acetylcysteine (NAC) Therapy Timeliness and Dosage Adjustments

4. Supratherapeutic and Modified-Release Formulations
Special Considerations and Management

5. Diagnostic Challenges in Unclear Exposure Cases

Chapter 7: Salicylate Poisoning

1. Altered Pharmacokinetics in Overdose

2. Clinical and Biochemical Monitoring

3. Metabolic and Neurological Effects

4. Urinary Alkalinization for Enhanced Elimination

5. Management of Chronic Salicylate Poisoning

Chapter 8: Antidiabetic Drugs

1. Insulin and Sulfonylurea Toxicity
Hypoglycemia and Prolonged Monitoring

2. Octreotide and Sulfonylurea Overdose

3. Glucose Management and Central Venous Access

4. Metformin Overdose and Lactic Acidosis

Chapter 9: Colchicine Poisoning

1. Life-Threatening Risks in Self-Poisoning

2. Diagnostic Indicators
Gastrointestinal Symptoms and Multi-Organ Failure

3. Aggressive Supportive Care Strategies

Chapter 10: Theophylline and Caffeine

1. Overview of Methylxanthine Toxicity

2. Severe Complications: Seizures and Cardiac Arrhythmias

3. Predictors of Toxicity
Hypokalaemia and Lactic Acidosis

4. Enhanced Elimination Techniques

Chapter 11: Iron Poisoning

1. Acute Iron Toxicity
Pathophysiology and Risk Factors

2. Dose-Dependent Toxicity of Elemental Iron
Local vs. Systemic Manifestations
Gastrointestinal Decontamination Techniques

3. Role of Intravenous Desferrioxamine in Severe Cases
Prognosis and Long-Term Complications

4. Iron Poisoning Management During Pregnancy

Chapter 12: Drugs of Abuse

1. Clinical Diagnosis and Supportive Care Principles

2. Opioid Overdose
Recognition and Naloxone Administration

3. Amphetamine Toxicity
Management and Complications

4. Cocaine-Induced Toxicities
Cardiac and Neurological Implications

5. Gamma-Hydroxybutyric Acid (GHB) Overdose
Clinical Management

6. Synthetic Psychoactive Substances
Challenges in Diagnosis

7. Prescription Drug Misuse
Trends and Interventions

8. Emergency Department Strategies for Overdose Cases

Chapter 13: Cyanide Poisoning

1. Mechanism of Cyanide Toxicity
A Metabolic Toxin
Rapid Onset Effects on the CNS, Respiratory, and Cardiovascular Systems

2. Diagnostic Markers
 Serum Lactate Levels
Immediate Resuscitation and Antidote Administration

3. Managing Cyanide Exposure in Smoke Inhalation Cases

Chapter 14: Hydrofluoric Acid Exposure

1. Recognizing the Hazard of Household HF Products
Clinical Features and Delayed Symptom Presentation

2. Emergency Decontamination and Irrigation Protocols
Advanced Calcium-Based Therapies for Persistent Pain

3. Systemic Toxicity
Electrolyte Imbalances and Cardiac Risks

4. Management of Severe HF Exposure Cases

Chapter 15: Pesticide Poisoning

1. Global Impact and Regional Trends in Acute Poisoning
Limitations of Current Toxicity Classification Systems

2. Role of Co-Formulants in Enhancing Toxicity Diagnosis

Clinical Features and Exposure History
Monitoring for Delayed Onset of Symptoms

3. Resuscitation and Supportive Care in Severe Cases
Preventing Secondary Contamination in Healthcare Settings

4. Anticholinesterase Pesticides
Use of Atropine and Pralidoxime

Chapter 16: Herbicides

1. Overview of Herbicide Toxicity and Challenges in Management

Paraquat Poisoning
High fatality rates and multi-organ failure
Lethal doses and absence of effective treatments

2. Glyphosate-Containing Herbicides
Toxic components and systemic effects
Supportive care for severe cases

3. Chlorophenoxy Herbicides
Mild toxicity and fatal risks
Increased toxicity with bromoxynil co-formulations

Chapter 17: Ethanol and Other Toxic Alcohols

1. Health Impact and Management Strategies

2. Ethanol Toxicity
Acute intoxication and chronic complications
CNS depressant effects and withdrawal risks
Wernicke Encephalopathy diagnosis and treatment

2. Toxic Alcohols
Methanol and ethylene glycol toxicity
Diagnosis using anion-gap and osmolar gap
Dialysis as a treatment option

Chapter 18: Carbon Monoxide Poisoning

1. Epidemiology and Sources of CO Poisoning

Leading cause of fatal poisoning in some regions
Common industrial and household sources

2. Neuropsychological and Long-Term Impact

3. Oxygen Therapy
Accelerating CO elimination
Debates on optimal oxygen administration methods

Chapter 19: Anticonvulsants

1. CNS and Cardiotoxic Effects of Overdose

2. Use of Activated Charcoal
Reducing toxicity duration in specific overdoses

3. Serum Drug Levels
Correlation with clinical toxicity

4. Extracorporeal Elimination for Severe Cases

5. Paradoxical Seizures

Chapter 20: Hymenoptera Stings

1. Epidemiology of Sting-Related Deaths

2. Allergic Reactions and Anaphylaxis Management

3. Venom Immunotherapy as Definitive Treatment

4. Risks of Multi-Organ Failure from Extensive Envenomation

5. Ant Stings and Rare Mass Envenomation Scenarios

Chapter 21: Toxidromes

1. Overview of Common Toxic Syndromes

2. Anticholinergic (Antimuscarinic) Toxic Syndrome
Pathophysiology and key medications causing ACTS

3. Serotonin Toxicity
Hallmark signs and diagnostic features
Drug interactions and exacerbating factors
Management strategies and clinical monitoring

Chapter 22: Chloroquine

1. Toxicity and Management of Chloroquine Overdose

2. High Mortality Risk and Rapid Cardiac Toxicity

3. Supportive Care and Adrenaline Administration

4. Role of Toxicology Consultation

5. Hospital Admission and Cardiac Monitoring

Chapter 23: Opioids

1. Toxicity Profiles and Treatment Approaches

2. Clinical Features of Opioid Toxicity
Respiratory depression, miosis, and altered consciousness

2. Naloxone Administration and Supportive Care

3. Additional Toxic Effects of Specific Opioids
Seizures (tramadol), QT prolongation (methadone), QRS widening (dextropropoxyphene)

4. Pediatric Exposure Risks

Chapter 24: Oral Anticoagulants

1. Overdose Management and Reversal Agents

2. Effects on INR and Dose-Dependent Toxicity

3. Role of Activated Charcoal in Reducing Absorption

4. Warfarin Overdose Guidelines

5. Reversal Agents and Their Efficacy
Prothrombinex-VF and idarucizumab

6. Acute Rivaroxaban Toxicity and Limited Harm Potential

List of Abbreviations

ACLS: Advanced Cardiac Life Support

ADME: Absorption, Distribution, Metabolism, and Excretion

AEDS: Antiepileptic Drugs

ALP: Alkaline Phosphatase

ALT: Alanine Aminotransferase

AST: Aspartate Aminotransferase

ATLS: Advanced Trauma Life Support

AV: Atrioventricular

BBB: Blood-Brain Barrier

BP: Blood Pressure

BUN: Blood Urea Nitrogen

CBC: Complete Blood Count

COX: Cyclooxygenase

CPK: Creatine Phosphokinase

CPR: Cardiopulmonary Resuscitation

CT: Computed Tomography

CVS: Cardiovascular System

DOAC: Direct Oral Anticoagulants

ECG: Electrocardiogram

ED: Emergency Department

EMS: Emergency Medical Services

GI: Gastrointestinal

ICU: Intensive Care Unit

IM: Intramuscular

INR: International Normalized Ratio

IV: Intravenous

LFT: Liver Function Test

LOC: Loss of Consciousness

LP: Lumbar Puncture

MI: Myocardial Infarction

MRI: Magnetic Resonance Imaging

NGT: Nasogastric Tube

NSAID: Nonsteroidal Anti-inflammatory Drug

PCC: Prothrombin Complex Concentrate

PEEP: Positive End-Expiratory Pressure

POC: Point-of-Care

PT: Prothrombin Time

PTE: Pulmonary Thromboembolism

PTT: Partial Thromboplastin Time

RRT: Renal Replacement Therapy

SOFA: Sequential Organ Failure Assessment

TCA: Tricyclic Antidepressants

VBG: Venous Blood Gas

VF: Ventricular Fibrillation

VT: Ventricular Tachycardia

WBC: White Blood Cell Count

Chapter 1
Comprehensive Approach to the Poisoned Patient

Key Considerations

1. Self-Poisoning as a Reflection of Underlying Issues: Intentional poisoning often signifies psychiatric, substance abuse, or social problems.

2. Diverse Clinical Presentations: Toxicity from drug overdoses presents varied symptoms affecting multiple organ systems.

3. Risk Assessment as a Predictor: Accurate assessment is vital for anticipating clinical progression and determining management strategies.

4. Emphasis on Supportive Care: Timely, appropriate supportive care is the cornerstone of poisoning management.

5. Gastrointestinal Decontamination: Considered based on risk-benefit analysis, it can be crucial even if delayed in select cases.

Management of Toxicology Cases: Techniques, Antidotes, and Evidence-Based Practices

Decontamination of the Gastrointestinal Tract

The primary goal of gastrointestinal decontamination is to prevent the absorption of toxic substances into the bloodstream. However, it should not be universally applied. The decision to employ decontamination methods should hinge on a risk-benefit analysis, considering the nature of the toxin, the quantity ingested, and the timing of presentation. Efforts to decontaminate should never take priority over resuscitation and supportive care.

Methods of Decontamination:

1. Gastric Emptying:

Techniques include the administration of emetics (e.g., syrup of ipecac) or gastric lavage.

Studies show limited efficacy unless performed within one hour of ingestion. Beyond this window, their effectiveness is negligible.

Routine use of gastric emptying has not demonstrated improved clinical outcomes except in select cases, such as unconscious patients presenting soon after ingestion.

2. Activated Charcoal (AC):

AC is the preferred decontamination method for most poisonings due to its ability to adsorb various pharmaceuticals and chemicals.

Materials that do not effectively bind to AC are listed in Box 25.1.7.

The efficacy of AC diminishes significantly over time, with the best results observed when administered within one hour of ingestion. Special scenarios such as massive overdoses, delayed-release formulations, or gastrointestinal motility issues may still benefit from AC use.

3. Whole-Bowel Irrigation (WBI):

WBI involves the administration of polyethylene glycol solution until rectal effluent is clear, typically over six hours.

Evidence supports its use in cases of slow-release drug ingestions, iron, lead, or drug-packet ingestion.

Contraindications include ileus, bowel obstruction, or unprotected airways.

Enhanced Elimination Techniques
Enhanced elimination methods are reserved for severe cases where standard supportive measures

are insufficient. Suitability depends on the pharmacokinetics of the toxin.

1. Multiple-Dose Activated Charcoal:

Enhances elimination through enterohepatic interruption or "gastrointestinal dialysis."

Effective for drugs like carbamazepine, theophylline, and phenobarbitone.

2. Urinary Alkalinization:

Facilitates the excretion of weak acids like salicylates by maintaining an alkaline urine pH.

3. Hemodialysis (HD) and Hemoperfusion (HP):

Indicated for toxins with low molecular weight, small distribution volumes, and slow endogenous clearance (e.g., ethylene glycol, methanol, lithium).

Antidotes in Toxicology

Antidotes are critical for managing specific toxicities but should be used judiciously, considering potential side effects. Table 25.1.4 outlines antidotes commonly used in emergency settings, including:

Physostigmine: For anticholinergic toxicity.

Hydroxocobalamin: For cyanide poisoning.

Naloxone: For opioid overdoses.

N-Acetylcysteine: For acetaminophen toxicity.

Clinical Investigations and Monitoring

Investigations should focus on diagnostics that directly influence patient management, including:

Electrocardiograms (ECG): To detect conduction defects in cardiotoxic poisonings.

Paracetamol Levels: To guide timely antidote administration.

Electrolytes and Renal Function Tests: For more severe intoxications.

Radiological studies, such as abdominal X-rays, may help identify ingested metals or drug packets. Advanced imaging like CT scans can exclude intracranial or abdominal pathologies in cases of altered mental status.

Disposition and Psychiatric Assessment

Stable patients without significant symptoms after 4-6 hours may be admitted to non-monitored beds or discharged.

Severe cases requiring supportive interventions necessitate intensive care monitoring.

Psychiatric evaluation is essential for cases of deliberate self-poisoning and should occur once the patient is medically stable.

Controversies in Practice
The routine application of gastric decontamination remains debated. Clinical decisions should prioritize patient safety and evidence-based practices, recognizing that universal protocols may not be appropriate.

This summary synthesizes key management principles, providing a comprehensive framework for managing toxicological emergencies based on current evidence and clinical guidelines.

6. Role of Antidotes: While rarely necessary, timely administration of antidotes can be life-saving in specific situations.

Introduction

Drug overdoses in adults predominantly occur as a result of self-poisoning, whether deliberate or recreational. In Australia, deliberate self-poisoning constitutes 1% to 5% of public hospital admissions. Effective management, primarily executed in emergency departments, requires clinicians to apply both general principles and context-specific strategies.

Importantly, acute overdose is often a transient manifestation of broader psychosocial issues. Recognizing this context aids in providing holistic care beyond the immediate toxicological event.

Key Clinical Presentations

Central Nervous System (CNS) Depression

Commonly resulting from substances such as alcohol, sedatives, opioids, or antidepressants, CNS depression can cause respiratory compromise due to ventilatory muscle failure or apnoea.

Respiratory Complications

Respiratory issues may stem from:

Aspiration: Common during periods of unconsciousness or seizures.

Pulmonary Oedema: Either cardiogenic or non-cardiogenic in origin.

Toxic Pulmonary Effects: Caused by specific agents like paraquat.

Cardiovascular Manifestations

These include a spectrum of effects, from tachycardia and bradycardia to conduction defects and severe arrhythmias.

Tachycardia: Often benign and attributed to sympathomimetics or anticholinergics.

Bradycardia: Less common but potentially life-threatening, associated with β-blockers or calcium channel blockers.

Hypertension and Hypotension: Hypertension is frequently linked to stimulant abuse, while hypotension may arise from myocardial depression, fluid loss, or vasodilation.

CNS Manifestations

Altered mental states, ranging from agitation and delirium to coma, are frequent.

Seizures: Toxic seizures are life-threatening, with common causes including tricyclic antidepressants, bupropion, and theophylline.

Thermal Dysregulation: Hypothermia often results from environmental exposure in unconscious patients, while hyperthermia is associated with serotonin syndrome or sympathomimetic overdose.

Pathophysiology and Dynamics

Poisoning is a dynamic process; symptoms and severity may fluctuate over time. Acute morbidity and mortality typically arise from effects on the cardiovascular, respiratory, or CNS systems. In rare cases, hepatic, renal, or metabolic derangements can be fatal.

Complications like aspiration, rhabdomyolysis, and renal failure are often consequences of secondary effects, such as prolonged immobility or severe agitation. Rapid intervention can mitigate these outcomes.

Assessment and Management

Risk Assessment

Risk assessment is pivotal in predicting clinical outcomes and guiding interventions. Key factors include:

Type and dose of substance.

Time has elapsed since ingestion.

Presenting clinical features.

Patient-specific factors (e.g., age, comorbidities).

History Taking

Collecting an accurate history is essential. If the patient is incapacitated, collateral information should be sought from family, paramedics, or other sources.

Physical Examination

Focused evaluation aims to:

Identify life-threatening complications.

Establish a baseline for monitoring.

Detecting toxidromes or alternative diagnoses.

Supportive Care and Monitoring

Airway and Ventilation: Maintain airway patency and provide oxygenation as needed.

Circulatory Support: Address hypotension or arrhythmias promptly.

Thermoregulation: Correct hypo- or hyperthermia.

Diagnostic Investigations

Universal Screening: Includes paracetamol levels and a 12-lead ECG.

Specialized Testing: May involve toxicology panels or imaging to refine diagnosis and risk assessment.

Decontamination and Antidote Use

Gastrointestinal Decontamination: Administered based on timing and risk-benefit considerations.

Antidotes: Reserved for specific toxins, such as naloxone for opioids or atropine for organophosphates.

Management of Toxicology Cases: Techniques, Antidotes, and Evidence-Based Practices

Decontamination of the Gastrointestinal Tract
The primary goal of gastrointestinal decontamination is to prevent the absorption of toxic substances into the bloodstream. However, it should not be universally applied. The decision to employ decontamination methods

should hinge on a risk-benefit analysis, considering the nature of the toxin, the quantity ingested, and the timing of presentation. Efforts to decontaminate should never take priority over resuscitation and supportive care.

Methods of Decontamination:

1. Gastric Emptying:

Techniques include the administration of emetics (e.g., syrup of ipecac) or gastric lavage.

Studies show limited efficacy unless performed within one hour of ingestion. Beyond this window, their effectiveness is negligible.

Routine use of gastric emptying has not demonstrated improved clinical outcomes except in select cases, such as unconscious patients presenting soon after ingestion.

2. Activated Charcoal (AC):

AC is the preferred decontamination method for most poisonings due to its ability to adsorb various pharmaceuticals and chemicals.

The efficacy of AC diminishes significantly over time, with the best results observed when administered within one hour of ingestion. Special scenarios such as massive overdoses, delayed-release formulations, or gastrointestinal motility issues may still benefit from AC use.

3. Whole-Bowel Irrigation (WBI):

WBI involves the administration of polyethylene glycol solution until rectal effluent is clear, typically over six hours.

Evidence supports its use in cases of slow-release drug ingestions, iron, lead, or drug-packet ingestion.

Contraindications include ileus, bowel obstruction, or unprotected airways.

Enhanced Elimination Techniques

Enhanced elimination methods are reserved for severe cases where standard supportive measures are insufficient. Suitability depends on the pharmacokinetics of the toxin.

1. Multiple-Dose Activated Charcoal:

Enhances elimination through enterohepatic interruption or "gastrointestinal dialysis."

Effective for drugs like carbamazepine, theophylline, and phenobarbitone.

2. Urinary Alkalinization:

Facilitates the excretion of weak acids like salicylates by maintaining an alkaline urine pH.

3. Hemodialysis (HD) and Hemoperfusion (HP):

Indicated for toxins with low molecular weight, small distribution volumes, and slow endogenous clearance (e.g., ethylene glycol, methanol, lithium).

Antidotes in Toxicology
Antidotes are critical for managing specific toxicities but should be used judiciously, considering potential side effects.

Physostigmine: For anticholinergic toxicity.

Hydroxocobalamin: For cyanide poisoning.

Naloxone: For opioid overdoses.

N-Acetylcysteine: For acetaminophen toxicity.

Clinical Investigations and Monitoring

Investigations should focus on diagnostics that directly influence patient management, including:

Electrocardiograms (ECG): To detect conduction defects in cardiotoxic poisonings.

Paracetamol Levels: To guide timely antidote administration.

Electrolytes and Renal Function Tests: For more severe intoxications.

Radiological studies, such as abdominal X-rays, may help identify ingested metals or drug packets. Advanced imaging like CT scans can exclude intracranial or abdominal pathologies in cases of altered mental status.

Disposition and Psychiatric Assessment

Stable patients without significant symptoms after 4-6 hours may be admitted to non-monitored beds or discharged.

Severe cases requiring supportive interventions necessitate intensive care monitoring.

Psychiatric evaluation is essential for cases of deliberate self-poisoning and should occur once the patient is medically stable.

Controversies in Practice

The routine application of gastric decontamination remains debated. Clinical decisions should prioritize patient safety and evidence-based practices, recognizing that universal protocols may not be appropriate.

References

1. McGrath J. An investigation into deliberate self-poisoning cases. Medical Journal of Australia, 1989;150:317–322.

2. Pond SM. Insights into prescription-related poisonings. Medical Journal of Australia, 1995;162:174–175.

3. Murray L, Little M, Pascu O, et al. Toxicology Handbook. 3rd edition. Sydney: Elsevier, 2015.

4. American Academy of Clinical Toxicology, European Association of Poisons Centres and Clinical Toxicologists. Position statement on the use of ipecac syrup. Journal of Toxicology: Clinical Toxicology, 2004;42:133–143.

5. Vale JA, Kulig K, American Academy of Clinical Toxicology, European Association of Poison Centres and Clinical Toxicologists. Position paper addressing gastric lavage. Journal of Toxicology: Clinical Toxicology, 2004;42:933–943.

6. Pond SM, Lewis-Driver DJ, Williams G. Evaluating gastric emptying during acute overdose: a randomized controlled trial. Medical Journal of Australia, 1995;163:345–349.

7. American Academy of Clinical Toxicology, European Association of Poisons Centres and Clinical Toxicologists. Position paper on the application of single-dose activated charcoal. Journal of Toxicology: Clinical Toxicology, 2005;43:61–87.

8. American Academy of Clinical Toxicology, European Association of Poisons Centres and Clinical Toxicologists. Position statement on the use of cathartics. Journal of Toxicology: Clinical Toxicology, 2004;42:243–253.

9. American Academy of Clinical Toxicology, European Association of Poisons Centres and Clinical Toxicologists. Position paper discussing whole bowel irrigation. Journal of Toxicology: Clinical Toxicology, 2004;24:843–854.

10. Chyka PA. A review of studies on multiple-dose activated charcoal and its role in enhancing systemic drug clearance in both animals and human subjects. Clinical Toxicology, 1995;33:399–404.

Chapter 2
Cardiovascular Drug Toxicity Management

Key Considerations

1. Life-Threatening Risks: Overdose of calcium channel blockers (CCBs), β-blockers, digoxin, and sodium channel blockers can result in severe, potentially fatal toxicity.

2. Management Strategy for CCBs and β-Blockers: The primary treatment involves aggressive circulatory support, including the early initiation of hyperinsulinemic euglycemic therapy, which is essential for reversing toxicity.

3. Delayed Onset in Slow-Release Formulations: Toxicity from slow-release CCBs may have a delayed onset, requiring special attention to timing in treatment.

4. Importance of Early Decontamination: For slow-release CCB overdoses, whole-bowel irrigation is a critical early step to reduce absorption and mitigate the severity of the overdose.

5. Sodium Channel Blocker Management: Treatment primarily involves sodium bicarbonate therapy and hyperventilation to manage sodium channel blocker toxicity.

6. Digoxin Toxicity: Early recognition of severe digoxin toxicity and the use of digoxin-specific antibody Fab fragments are lifesaving.

7. Clonidine Poisoning: Management remains mainly supportive, addressing symptoms and vital organ support.

8. Intravenous Lipid Emulsion (ILE) Therapy: ILE is reserved for severe local anesthetic toxicity and is not considered standard treatment for other drug overdoses.

Calcium Channel Blockers (CCBs) and β-Blockers: Overview and Toxicity Management

Introduction CCBs and β-blockers are commonly used cardiovascular drugs, but overdose can lead to severe and potentially fatal effects. Both types of overdose present with similar clinical manifestations, primarily impacting cardiac function. While CCB and β-blocker overdose management shares many similarities, understanding the specific pharmacokinetics, pathophysiology, and clinical features is crucial for effective treatment.

Pharmacokinetics of CCBs and β-Blockers

CCBs are rapidly absorbed from the gastrointestinal tract, with effects generally occurring within 30 minutes. However, the onset of symptoms may be delayed in the case of slow-release formulations.

β-Blockers, such as propranolol, are absorbed rapidly, with peak effects typically observed within 1 to 4 hours. The pharmacokinetic profiles vary based on the specific agent and its lipid solubility, which influences central nervous system (CNS) toxicity.

In overdose scenarios, all CCBs can cause prolonged effects, with amlodipine having a notably longer half-life (30–50 hours), requiring extended monitoring. Slow-release forms of both verapamil and diltiazem can cause delayed toxic effects, requiring careful timing in management.

Pathophysiology

CCBs inhibit the entry of calcium into cells, leading to reduced myocardial contractility and slowed conduction through the sinus and atrioventricular (AV) nodes. This results in hypotension, bradycardia, and a risk of severe arrhythmias.

β-Blockers block β1 and β2 receptors, leading to decreased heart rate, contractility, and conduction velocity, thereby reducing cardiac output. Some β-blockers, such as propranolol, can also affect myocardial sodium channels, which exacerbates conduction defects.

Clinical Features of Toxicity

CCBs: Symptoms of toxicity vary depending on the drug and dose but often include bradycardia, hypotension, shock, and altered mental status. With slow-release formulations, symptom onset can be delayed, complicating early intervention.

β-Blockers: Severe toxicity can result in bradycardia, hypotension, heart block, and ventricular arrhythmias. Symptoms may include CNS effects such as confusion and seizures, especially with more lipid-soluble agents like propranolol. Toxicity is more likely to manifest within 6 hours of ingestion.

Clinical Investigation and Monitoring

ECG: The electrocardiogram (ECG) is essential in diagnosing and monitoring conduction defects, arrhythmias, and other cardiovascular effects. Specific changes like prolonged PR intervals, QRS prolongation, and heart block should prompt closer evaluation.

Serum Drug Levels: Serum drug concentrations are not always useful in managing toxicity; therefore, clinical evaluation and symptomatic management are paramount.

Electrolyte and Glucose Monitoring: Patients with severe toxicity should have continuous monitoring of electrolytes, particularly calcium, and blood glucose, as these can be impacted by the overdose and treatment interventions.

Treatment Approaches

Calcium Channel Blockers and β-Blockers

Circulatory Support: The cornerstone of treatment for both CCB and β-blocker toxicity is to restore adequate tissue perfusion and maintain cardiac output. Initial management involves:

Airway and Ventilatory Support: Ensuring oxygenation and ventilation are critical in maintaining organ function.

Intravenous Fluids: Aggressive fluid resuscitation is necessary to address hypotension and shock.

Specific Therapies:

Hyperinsulinemic Euglycemic Therapy: This technique has been shown to improve myocardial function and can be particularly effective in managing both CCB and β-blocker toxicity.

Atropine and Glucagon: In β-blocker overdose, glucagon can reverse some of the negative inotropic and chronotropic effects, while atropine may be used to address bradycardia.

Calcium Salts: In severe CCB toxicity, intravenous calcium may be used to counteract the calcium blockade in the myocardium, helping to restore normal contractility.

Decontamination: In cases of significant overdose, whole-bowel irrigation is recommended, particularly for slow-release CCBs. This procedure helps to reduce further absorption and mitigate the severity of the overdose.

Sodium Channel Blockers and Digoxin

Sodium Channel Blocker Toxicity: Sodium bicarbonate administration and hyperventilation are key to managing toxicity, as they help to reverse the effects on cardiac conduction.

Digoxin Toxicity: Recognizing severe toxicity early and administering digoxin-specific antibody Fab fragments is a lifesaving intervention.

Clonidine Poisoning

Supportive Care: Most cases of clonidine poisoning require only supportive care, such as fluid management and close monitoring, although naloxone may be helpful in some cases due to its opioid-like effects.

Intravenous Lipid Emulsion (ILE) Therapy

Use in Local Anesthetic Toxicity: ILE therapy is recommended primarily for severe cases of local anesthetic toxicity, but it is not considered standard for managing other drug overdoses.

Treatment of Digoxin Toxicity

Early Detection and Management The key to optimal outcomes in digoxin toxicity is early recognition. For acute overdose, patients should be managed in a monitored setting equipped for resuscitation, where immediate attention to airway, breathing, and circulation may be necessary. Establish intravenous access and send blood for urgent electrolyte and digoxin concentration tests. Activated charcoal, which binds to digoxin, should be administered if the patient is able to tolerate it, although repeated vomiting may complicate its use.

Chronic Toxicity Management In cases of chronic digoxin toxicity with minimal symptoms, management may require only observation, cessation of digoxin, and correction of hypokalemia and hypomagnesemia. Additionally, treating underlying conditions contributing to toxicity is essential. If the patient exhibits symptoms like brady-tachy arrhythmias causing hemodynamic instability, or increased automaticity with cardiac and gastrointestinal symptoms, digoxin-specific antibody therapy may be necessary, particularly for those with renal impairment (creatinine clearance <30 mL/min).

Digoxin-Specific Antibody Therapy (Digoxin Fab) The specific antidote for digoxin toxicity is the Fab fragments of digoxin-specific antibodies. These antibodies, derived from sheep immunoglobulin, bind to digoxin in the bloodstream, reducing its activity. The therapeutic effect is typically seen within 20 to 30 minutes of administration. The Fab-digoxin complexes are excreted in the urine. A dosage of 40 mg (1 vial) of digoxin Fab binds 0.5 mg of digoxin. While prior dosing recommendations suggested an equimolar dose to stabilize severe toxicity, recent studies suggest staggered dosing over 24 to 48 hours based on ECG changes and clinical response.

Clinical Response and Monitoring In cases of chronic toxicity, digoxin Fab is less effective, particularly in managing arrhythmias. The typical response to the antidote in these cases includes a significant reduction in free digoxin levels, although heart rate changes may be modest. Smaller hospitals should maintain at least 2 vials of digoxin Fab, ensuring readiness for any acute situation.

Disposition For acute overdoses, patients should be closely monitored for 24 to 48 hours. Those requiring further treatment with digoxin Fab should be observed for electrolyte imbalances, particularly hypokalemia. Any intentional ingestions should also prompt psychiatric evaluation prior to discharge. For patients with mild chronic toxicity, management may include cessation of digoxin therapy, with discharge possible if no significant arrhythmias, electrolyte disturbances, or renal failure are present.

Clonidine Overdose

Introduction and Pharmacokinetics Clonidine, initially developed as a nasal decongestant, is a central α2-adrenergic agonist used primarily for hypertension, ADHD, and withdrawal symptoms. It is highly absorbed with near 100% bioavailability, reaching peak plasma concentrations within 1 to 3 hours, with a half-life of 6 to 24 hours, excreted primarily unchanged by the kidneys.

Pathophysiology Clonidine acts on the vasomotor center in the medulla oblongata to reduce sympathetic outflow, leading to a reduction in cardiac output and a slowing of heart rate. At higher doses, it may paradoxically cause initial hypertension due to its partial α1-adrenergic agonist effect.

Clinical Features Overdose symptoms typically manifest within 30 minutes and include CNS depression, bradycardia, transient hypertension, hypotension, coma, seizures, miosis, respiratory depression, and hypothermia. Children are particularly vulnerable to severe CNS depression and respiratory issues, while adults may experience persistent bradycardia for up to 48 hours.

Investigations An ECG is essential to monitor bradycardia and potential conduction defects.

Treatment Management is primarily supportive, with intravenous fluids to address hypotension. The use of atropine and naloxone has been reported, though results vary. In rare cases, vasopressors may be required. While hypertension is often brief and self-limiting, naloxone's role in reversing CNS depression or bradycardia is debated.

Disposition Patients should be observed in the hospital until they are asymptomatic, with bradycardia resolved. Continuous cardiac monitoring is not necessary unless the patient remains symptomatic.

Class 1C Antiarrhythmic Overdose

Introduction Class 1C antiarrhythmics, such as flecainide and propafenone, block sodium channels, leading to prolonged QRS duration and potential cardiovascular collapse in overdose situations. These agents are used for treating supraventricular tachycardia and ventricular arrhythmias.

Pharmacokinetics Flecainide has high oral bioavailability, with effects manifesting within 30 to 60 minutes and a half-life of 7 to 23 hours. Ingestions of 800 mg or more are considered life-threatening. Propafenone has a similar pharmacokinetic profile.

Clinical Features Overdose symptoms typically appear within 30 minutes to 2 hours and include nausea, vomiting, hypotension, bradycardia, AV block, tachyarrhythmias, and in severe cases, coma or seizures. Fatalities often occur within 3 to 15 hours due to rapid cardiovascular collapse.

Investigations An ECG is crucial to monitor QRS duration, conduction defects, and the QT interval. A QRS width greater than 120 ms is the hallmark of toxicity.

Treatment Supportive care is the primary approach, with inotropic support, gastrointestinal decontamination, and sodium bicarbonate therapy. Sodium bicarbonate helps by alkalinizing the plasma to reverse sodium channel blockade, especially in patients with broad-complex arrhythmias and hypotension. Repeated doses of sodium bicarbonate may be necessary if symptoms recur. In extreme cases, transcutaneous pacing or ECMO may be considered for refractory arrhythmias.

Disposition Patients with normal ECGs and no symptoms 4 hours post-ingestion are unlikely to develop toxicity. Symptomatic patients should be admitted to a monitored setting for ongoing observation.

Chapter 3
Antipsychotic Drugs

Key Considerations

1. Antipsychotics can lead to a range of adverse effects at therapeutic doses, which may hinder patient adherence to treatment.

2. Extrapyramidal symptoms (EPS) are less frequent with second-generation antipsychotics compared to first-generation agents.

3. Clozapine usage is associated with serious side effects like agranulocytosis and myocarditis, necessitating rigorous monitoring.

4. Antipsychotic overdose primarily results in central nervous system (CNS) depression and cardiovascular complications.

5. Amisulpride may cause QT interval prolongation, raising the risk of torsades de pointes.

6. The treatment of antipsychotic overdose is mainly supportive.

7. Neuroleptic malignant syndrome (NMS) is a rare but severe reaction that can be fatal without timely intervention.

Introduction

Antipsychotics represent a diverse group of medications, with their use dating back to the 1950s, when chlorpromazine was first introduced for the treatment of schizophrenia. The early-generation, or 'typical,' antipsychotics were linked to numerous adverse effects, especially movement disorders like extrapyramidal symptoms (EPS). These drugs also demonstrated limited efficacy in addressing the negative symptoms of schizophrenia. In response, second-generation or 'atypical' antipsychotics were developed in the late 1980s. These newer agents generally present with fewer movement-related side effects and are more effective in treating the negative symptoms of schizophrenia while still managing acute psychosis. As a result, second-generation antipsychotics have largely replaced first-generation drugs as the primary treatment for schizophrenia and other psychotic disorders.

Over the past three decades, there has been an increase in antipsychotic prescriptions in Australia, including for off-label indications. This has also led to a rise in self-poisoning cases. Despite the perception that second-generation antipsychotics like quetiapine and olanzapine are safer, overdose cases involving these drugs have not led to a reduction in morbidity or in-hospital mortality rates.

Pharmacology

Antipsychotic medications can be classified in various ways, including as typical or atypical agents, by their chemical structure, or based on their neuroreceptor binding properties. All antipsychotics exert their therapeutic effects primarily by antagonizing dopamine D2 receptors in the mesolimbic system. Early-generation antipsychotics were categorized as either high- or low-potency based on their D2 receptor affinity. However, antagonism at other D2 receptor sites can contribute to numerous adverse effects, such as movement disorders (when D2 receptors are blocked in the nigrostriatal pathway), negative symptoms of schizophrenia (when blocked in the mesocortical area), and elevated prolactin secretion (when blocked in the anterior pituitary, leading to conditions like gynecomastia and galactorrhea). Blockage of D2 receptors in the hypothalamus can also disrupt temperature regulation, contributing to hypo- or hyperthermia and potentially leading to neuroleptic malignant syndrome (NMS).

Second-generation antipsychotics primarily derive their therapeutic efficacy from antagonism at various serotonin (5-HT) receptors. Specifically, antagonism at the 5-HT2A receptor is thought to both enhance the treatment of negative symptoms of schizophrenia and reduce the likelihood of EPS. Agents with a higher affinity for muscarinic M1 and M2 receptors, such as olanzapine and quetiapine, can lead to anticholinergic toxicity, manifesting as agitation, delirium, and peripheral effects. Drugs with greater anticholinergic effects typically induce fewer extrapyramidal symptoms. High-affinity antagonism at histamine H1 receptors can cause sedation and, to a lesser extent, hypotension. Blocking the α1-adrenergic receptor may lead to hypotension, as seen with clozapine and quetiapine.

First-generation antipsychotics may also block sodium channels, which, in overdose situations, can slow cardiac conduction, widen the QRS complex, and impair myocardial contractility. Additionally, they may inhibit potassium channels, leading to delayed repolarization and QT prolongation.

While antipsychotics vary in their pharmacokinetic profiles, they are generally well-absorbed after oral administration, with peak plasma concentrations typically occurring within 2 to 6 hours. Their lipophilic nature, large volumes of distribution, and extensive protein binding contribute to their efficacy. Most are metabolized in the liver, with some having active metabolites.

Clinical Effects

Adverse Effects
Adverse effects of antipsychotics can be dose-related or idiosyncratic, with some effects appearing later in treatment.

Extrapyramidal Symptoms (EPS)
EPS refers to a range of disorders involving abnormal neuromuscular activity, often leading

to patient distress and poor treatment adherence. The four most common EPS include acute dystonia, akathisia, parkinsonism, and tardive dyskinesia. While the first three are usually reversible, tardive dyskinesia is irreversible and typically emerges after prolonged treatment (months to years).

Acute Dystonia: Characterized by involuntary muscle contractions, typically affecting the face, head, neck, or limbs. Laryngeal involvement, although rare, can be life-threatening. This condition usually develops within hours of drug exposure but may be delayed.

Akathisia: A subjective feeling of restlessness, often misattributed to the underlying psychiatric disorder. It may result in an inability to remain still.

Drug-Induced Parkinsonism: Resembling idiopathic Parkinson's disease, this condition involves rigidity and bradykinesia, though tremors may be less noticeable. It is more common in older patients and those on high-potency agents.

Tardive Dyskinesia: Involuntary, repetitive movements, most often involving facial and oral muscles but potentially affecting limbs and the trunk. This condition arises after extended antipsychotic use and is resistant to treatment.

Cardiovascular Effects
Antipsychotics can lead to tachycardia, postural hypotension, and ECG changes, including QRS and QT prolongation. These cardiovascular effects are often due to α1-adrenergic blockade and direct myocardial depression. Postural hypotension can occur due to vasodilatation.

Seizures
While all antipsychotics can lower the seizure threshold, seizures are rare unless the patient has underlying risk factors such as organic brain disease or epilepsy.

Metabolic Syndromes

Long-term use of many antipsychotics is linked to the development of metabolic syndrome, which includes weight gain, dyslipidemia, hypertension, and impaired glucose tolerance. These effects can reduce patient compliance and increase the risk of cardiovascular diseases and type II diabetes. Drugs like olanzapine and clozapine are particularly associated with these metabolic disturbances.

Neuroleptic Malignant Syndrome (NMS)

NMS is a rare but life-threatening condition that can occur with any antipsychotic medication. It is characterized by hyperthermia, muscle rigidity, autonomic dysfunction, and altered mental status. Early diagnosis and prompt management are crucial to prevent mortality.

Clozapine

Clozapine is a second-generation antipsychotic that requires careful monitoring due to its association with serious adverse effects, such as agranulocytosis and myocarditis. These conditions should be considered if a patient taking clozapine suddenly becomes ill.

Overdose Management

Overdose of antipsychotics typically leads to CNS depression and cardiovascular effects. Symptoms can range from lethargy and somnolence to coma and seizures, with potential impairment of airway reflexes, requiring intensive care. Many antipsychotics, especially those with strong anticholinergic properties, can induce delirium and peripheral toxicity. Tachycardia and hypotension are common cardiovascular symptoms, often due to α1-adrenergic blockade and anticholinergic effects. ECG changes may include QRS prolongation and QT prolongation.

Amisulpride

Overdose of amisulpride can cause sedation, bradycardia, hypotension, and QT prolongation. In severe cases, torsades de pointes may occur. The onset of cardiotoxicity can be delayed, and QT prolongation may persist for hours.

Chlorpromazine
Large overdoses (greater than 5 g) of chlorpromazine can cause significant CNS depression and hypotension. QT prolongation may also be observed.

Clozapine
Acute overdose with clozapine leads to CNS depression, which is more severe in clozapine-naïve individuals, who may require intubation. Seizures and hypersalivation are commonly observed, and while agranulocytosis does not result from a single overdose, it remains a serious concern in long-term use.

Haloperidol
Overdose with haloperidol often results in sedation and EPS. It is also associated with QT

prolongation and arrhythmias, particularly with large doses or intravenous administration.

Olanzapine
The clinical effects of olanzapine overdose typically emerge within 6 hours and include sedation and anticholinergic effects, with agitation and drowsiness possibly requiring intubation. Tachycardia is common, but significant ECG changes are rare.

Quetiapine
Overdose of quetiapine can lead to sedation, tachycardia, and hypotension, though severe complications are relatively uncommon.

References

1. Balit CR, Isbister GK, Hackett LP, et al. Quetiapine overdose: A case series. Ann Emerg Med. 2003;42:751-758.

2. Berling I, Buckley NA, Isbister GK. The antipsychotic dilemma: Shifts in prescriptions

and overdose rates without improved safety. Br J Clin Pharmacol. 2016;82:249-254.

3. Hawkins DJ, Unwin P. Severe hypotension following adrenaline infusions in massive quetiapine overdose: A paradoxical response. Crit Care Resusc. 2008;10:320-322.

4. Isbister GK, Balit CR, Kilham HA. Antipsychotic poisoning in young children. Drug Safety. 2005;28:1029-1034.

5. Isbister GK, Balit CR, Macleod D, Duffull SB. Amisulpride overdose: A common cause of QT prolongation and torsades de pointes. J Clin Psychopharmacol. 2010;30:391-395.

6. Juurlink DN. Antipsychotics. In: Nelson LS, Levin NA, Howland MA, eds. Goldfrank's Toxicologic Emergencies. 9th ed. New York: McGraw-Hill; 2010:1003-1015.

7. Levine M, Ruhn A-M. Overdose of atypical antipsychotics: Clinical manifestations,

mechanisms of toxicity, and management. CNS Drugs. 2012;26:601-611.

8. Minns AB, Clark RF. Toxicology and overdose of atypical antipsychotics. J Emerg Med. 2012;43:906-913.

9. Page CB, Calver LA, Isbister GK. Risperidone overdose: Extrapyramidal effects without cardiac toxicity. J Clin Psychopharmacol. 2010;30:387-390.

Chapter 4
Antidepressant Drugs

Key Considerations

1. Overdose of tricyclic antidepressants (TCAs) can lead to severe cardiovascular toxicity, seizures, coma, and death.

2. Sodium bicarbonate is the treatment of choice for TCA-induced cardiotoxicity.

3. Selective serotonin reuptake inhibitors (SSRIs) typically cause mild symptoms in overdose but may lead to significant serotonin toxicity when taken in very large amounts or in combination with other serotonergic agents.

4. While SSRIs rarely cause cardiovascular issues, citalopram and escitalopram are known to cause QT prolongation and torsades de pointes.

5. Selective noradrenaline reuptake inhibitors can lead to serotonin and sympathomimetic toxicity, with the potential for delayed seizures and cardiovascular issues after significant overdoses.

6. Overdose of monoamine oxidase inhibitors (MAOIs) can lead to delayed severe sympathomimetic stimulation, requiring intensive care management.

Introduction:
The severity of clinical toxicity after an overdose (OD) of antidepressant medications in Australia varies depending on the drug class. Toxic effects are typically dose-dependent and affect multiple organ systems. Cardiovascular and neurological manifestations, particularly in severe cases, can be life-threatening. Early risk assessment and aggressive supportive care are crucial for improving outcomes.

Tricyclic Antidepressants (TCAs):

While TCAs are effective for treating depression, they are more toxic in overdose compared to other antidepressant classes. Serious toxicity, including death, typically occurs with doses greater than 10 mg/kg in adults and 5 mg/kg in children. Among the TCAs available in Australia, dothiepin is linked to the highest toxicity. Cardiovascular dysfunction and coma typically develop quickly after significant ingestion, and the prognosis heavily depends on early airway management, sodium bicarbonate administration, and intensive care support.

Pharmacology of TCAs:
TCAs have a tertiary amine structure that interacts with various receptors throughout the body. These interactions contribute to both therapeutic and toxic effects.

CNS Effects: TCAs inhibit the reuptake of serotonin and noradrenaline in the central nervous system, which is central to their antidepressant effects. However, these same properties can also contribute to serotonin toxicity in overdose situations.

Cardiovascular Effects: TCAs block cardiac sodium channels, impairing sodium conductance, leading to membrane instability, QRS prolongation, arrhythmias, and impaired myocardial contractility.

Sedation and CNS Depression: TCAs also bind to histamine receptors, leading to CNS depression and sedation, which may result in coma.

Anticholinergic Effects: By antagonizing muscarinic receptors, TCAs can cause tachycardia, agitation, and urinary retention.

Vasodilation: Antagonism of α1-adrenergic receptors can result in peripheral vasodilation.

Other Effects: TCAs can also affect potassium, chloride, and GABA receptors, contributing to their diverse toxic profile.

TCAs are well absorbed after ingestion and are metabolized by the liver. They are highly protein-bound, lipophilic, and widely distributed throughout the body, with long half-lives (10 to 81 hours), which can be prolonged further in overdose situations.

Clinical Features of TCA Overdose:
The most common symptoms of TCA overdose include CNS depression, which can range from agitation and delirium to coma, and sinus tachycardia, typically developing within 1 to 2 hours of ingestion. These are accompanied by anticholinergic effects such as dry mouth, blurred vision, and urinary retention. The overdose also leads to significant cardiovascular effects, including arrhythmias, hypotension, and asystole. Seizures, caused by sodium channel blockade and subsequent acidosis, further exacerbate cardiovascular toxicity. Severe cases can lead to prolonged anticholinergic delirium, which may last up to 48 hours.

Clinical Investigations:
A 12-lead ECG is a critical diagnostic tool for predicting the severity of TCA toxicity. Key markers include QRS duration, with a prolonged QRS (>100 ms) being linked to worse outcomes, such as the need for intubation, seizures, or arrhythmias. A QRS duration over 160 ms can predict ventricular arrhythmias. Additionally, abnormalities such as a rightward frontal plane QRS vector and a positive R wave amplitude in lead aVR are sensitive indicators of TCA toxicity.

Although measuring plasma TCA concentrations is possible, it does not reliably correlate with clinical symptoms, making ECG and clinical evaluation more valuable in assessing overdose severity.

Treatment of TCA Overdose:
Aggressive supportive care is essential for patients who have ingested potentially toxic doses of TCAs. Early endotracheal intubation

should be performed if there is any decrease in consciousness, as hypoxia can exacerbate toxicity. Activated charcoal should be administered within 1 hour of ingestion, provided the airway is protected. For patients with severe toxicity, including those requiring intubation, activated charcoal may be given up to 4 hours after ingestion.

Sodium bicarbonate is the mainstay of treatment for TCA-induced cardiotoxicity. It should be administered early, especially in cases with QRS prolongation, arrhythmias, or hypotension unresponsive to fluids. Sodium bicarbonate is a hypertonic solution that competitively inhibits sodium channel blockade, improving cardiac conduction and reducing the concentration of TCAs that can exert toxic effects.

In addition to sodium bicarbonate, treatments for arrhythmias such as hypertonic saline (3% sodium chloride) and lignocaine may be considered. Antiarrhythmic agents like class 1a, 1c, and class III agents, as well as β-blockers and calcium channel blockers, should be avoided. Hypotension should be treated with intravenous fluids, and norepinephrine may be used for persistent hypotension.

Disposition:
Patients without CNS depression and with a normal ECG 6 hours after ingesting a potentially toxic dose of a TCA may be safely discharged. However, those showing signs of significant toxicity, such as abnormal ECG findings, should be admitted to an intensive care unit for continuous monitoring.

Monoamine Oxidase Inhibitors (MAOIs):
Pharmacology:
MAOIs, including irreversible non-selective drugs like phenelzine and tranylcypromine, and the reversible selective inhibitor moclobemide, increase CNS concentrations of neurotransmitters such as serotonin, noradrenaline, dopamine, and adrenaline. Irreversible MAOIs cause prolonged toxicity, lasting days, as the enzyme must be

resynthesized. In contrast, reversible MAOIs are less toxic, although they may still cause severe serotonin toxicity when combined with other serotonergic drugs.

MAOIs are well absorbed orally, cross the blood-brain barrier, and are metabolized by the liver. Peak concentrations typically occur within 2 to 3 hours after ingestion.

Clinical Features of MAOI Overdose:
Overdose with irreversible MAOIs initially manifests as peripheral sympathomimetic stimulation and CNS excitation. Symptoms typically begin 6 to 12 hours post-ingestion but can be delayed up to 24 hours. Early symptoms include nausea, headache, palpitations, agitation, and restlessness. As toxicity progresses, signs such as tachycardia, hyperreflexia, mydriasis, fasciculations, and nystagmus appear. Severe cases may progress to hypertensive crises, seizures, and potentially life-threatening arrhythmias.

25.4 Antidepressant Drugs

Overview of Toxicity: Antidepressant drugs, specifically Selective Serotonin Reuptake Inhibitors (SSRIs) and Serotonin-Norepinephrine Reuptake Inhibitors (SNRIs), can cause serious adverse effects, including cardiovascular dysfunction, multiorgan failure, seizures, and muscle rigidity. These side effects are more common with overdoses (OD).

SSRIs: Citalopram and Escitalopram Toxicity

Mechanism of Toxicity: Citalopram and escitalopram prolonged myocardial cell depolarization by inhibiting the efflux of potassium channels in myocardial cells. As a result, overdose of these medications can cause significant QT interval prolongation and may trigger torsades de pointes, a life-threatening arrhythmia.

Management: In the event of an overdose, activated charcoal is useful within one hour of massive SSRI ingestion (specifically, greater than 300 mg of escitalopram or 600 mg of citalopram), as it reduces the risk of prolonged QT intervals. Supportive care remains the cornerstone of treatment. Patients exhibiting mild to moderate serotonin excess symptoms generally benefit from benzodiazepines to alleviate symptoms. In severe cases, serotonin 2A receptor antagonists, such as cyproheptadine or chlorpromazine, may be used.

For serious cases of serotonin toxicity, admission to an intensive care unit (ICU) is often required. Patients with ingestion amounts over 1000 mg of citalopram or 400 mg of escitalopram (or lower doses if activated charcoal has not been administered within 4 hours) should undergo regular ECG monitoring. Cardiac monitoring should continue for at least 12 hours or until the QT interval normalizes.

Combined Serotonin and Norepinephrine Reuptake Inhibitors (SNRIs)

Pharmacology: SNRIs, such as duloxetine, reboxetine, venlafaxine, and desvenlafaxine, inhibit the reuptake of both serotonin and norepinephrine in the central nervous system. This results in more rapid therapeutic effects compared to SSRIs. They are absorbed quickly after oral ingestion and metabolized in the liver. Desvenlafaxine and venlafaxine are available only in modified-release formulations in Australia.

Toxicity and Clinical Features: Overdose with SNRIs increases synaptic concentrations of both serotonin and norepinephrine, resulting in a combination of serotonin toxicity and sympathomimetic toxidrome. Symptoms may include tachycardia, tremors, nausea, vomiting, dizziness, and agitation, which can be delayed with modified-release formulations. Venlafaxine overdose can cause serotonin syndrome in about 30% of cases, and higher doses are associated with a significant risk of seizures, with a dose-dependent relationship. Severe cardiovascular complications, including QRS and QT prolongation, may occur, especially with massive overdoses (e.g., >8 g of venlafaxine). Takotsubo cardiomyopathy has been observed even with therapeutic doses, particularly with venlafaxine and desvenlafaxine.

Management: Large ingestions of SNRIs necessitate monitoring in a facility with cardiac monitoring and seizure management capabilities. Activated charcoal should be considered for ingestion within 1 hour for standard-release formulations and 4 hours for modified-release formulations. Benzodiazepines are administered to control agitation, and seizures typically require intravenous benzodiazepines. In cases of severe toxicity, sodium bicarbonate should be used to treat QRS prolongation.

For ingestion of >5 g of venlafaxine, patients should be monitored for at least 24 hours due to the risk of delayed seizures.

Mirtazapine

Pharmacology and Toxicity: Mirtazapine is a tetracyclic antidepressant that enhances serotonin and norepinephrine release by antagonizing CNS α-receptors, specifically α2. It does not act as a serotonin reuptake inhibitor and has sedative properties due to its antihistamine receptor activity. Toxicity is relatively mild, with symptoms limited to sedation, tachycardia, and hypertension. Severe complications, such as seizures or cardiovascular toxicity, are rare.

Management: Treatment is supportive, as the toxicity is usually minor.

Bupropion

Pharmacology: Bupropion is a unicyclic antidepressant with a structure resembling amphetamines. It inhibits the reuptake of dopamine, with a lesser effect on norepinephrine and serotonin. It is metabolized to hydroxyl-bupropion, which has a long half-life, contributing to the extended effects of overdose. In Australia, it is available as a modified-release formulation.

Toxicity: Bupropion overdose poses a high risk of seizures, often occurring 6 to 8 hours after ingestion (up to 16 hours in some cases). Doses >9 g increase the risk significantly, with 100% of cases exhibiting seizures. Other symptoms may include tachycardia, hypertension, nausea, and tremors. Arrhythmias, including QT and QRS prolongation, have been reported in high doses, and fatalities have occurred following massive overdoses.

Management: Supportive care is essential, with a focus on managing seizures and cardiovascular instability. Intravenous benzodiazepines should be administered to control seizures and agitation. QRS prolongation can be treated with sodium bicarbonate, and hypotension should be managed with intravenous fluids. Activated charcoal should be administered within 4 hours of ingestion in cooperative patients.

Disposition:

Patients without seizures, agitation, or significant cardiovascular instability, and with a normal ECG 16 hours post-bupropion overdose, can be safely discharged. However, those with persistent symptoms should be admitted to an ICU for further management.

References:

1. Whyte IM, et al. Relative toxicity of venlafaxine and selective serotonin reuptake inhibitors in overdose. QJM. 2003;96:369-374.

2. Bateman ND. Tricyclic antidepressant poisoning: central nervous system effects and management. Toxicol Rev. 2005;24:181-186.

3. Thanacoody HKR, et al. Tricyclic antidepressant poisoning–cardiovascular toxicity. Toxicol Rev. 2005;24:205-214.

4. Caravati EM. The electrocardiogram as a diagnostic discriminator for acute tricyclic antidepressant poisoning. J Toxicol Clin Toxicol. 1999;37(1):113-115.

5. Bradberry SM, et al. Management of the cardiovascular complications of tricyclic antidepressant toxicity: role of sodium bicarbonate. Toxicol Rev. 2005;24:195-204.

Chapter 5
Lithium

Key Considerations

1. Chronic Lithium Toxicity:

Chronic lithium toxicity is a serious condition that can result in significant morbidity and mortality if diagnosis and treatment are delayed.

Early recognition of lithium toxicity in patients on lithium therapy is essential. A serum lithium level test should be conducted promptly.

Impaired renal function is the primary cause of chronic lithium toxicity, necessitating correction of the underlying factors.

Neurological symptoms are a hallmark of chronic toxicity, which may include tremors, ataxia, and confusion.

Serum lithium levels alone do not correlate well with the clinical severity of toxicity or central nervous system (CNS) involvement.

2. Acute Lithium Overdose:

Acute overdose in individuals not previously treated with lithium generally has a more favorable prognosis unless ingestion is massive (>25 g).

Common symptoms include nausea, vomiting, and diarrhea, which are due to gastrointestinal irritation. These symptoms can lead to dehydration and electrolyte imbalance.

Although serum lithium levels are useful in assessing treatment progress, they may not reflect the severity of clinical symptoms.

3. Acute-on-Chronic Lithium Toxicity:

Patients with both acute overdose and chronic lithium use are at a higher risk of neurotoxicity due to the cumulative lithium burden in the body.

Close monitoring for signs of neurotoxicity is crucial in these cases.

4. Hemodialysis for Lithium Elimination:

Hemodialysis can expedite lithium elimination, particularly in patients with impaired renal function or neurotoxicity in chronic toxicity.

It is rarely needed for acute lithium overdose in individuals with normal kidney function but may be required if renal function declines or in cases of severe intoxication.

Introduction

Lithium, a metal with the lowest molecular weight, is most commonly used in the form of lithium carbonate for the treatment of bipolar disorder and other psychiatric conditions. It is available in both immediate-release and sustained-release formulations. Despite its widespread use, lithium has a narrow therapeutic index, which increases the risk of toxicity with prolonged use or acute overdose.

Pharmacokinetics

Lithium is absorbed rapidly and almost completely following oral administration, with peak serum concentrations occurring 2 to 4 hours post-ingestion. For sustained-release formulations, absorption is delayed, especially in the case of overdose.

Once absorbed, lithium is redistributed from the bloodstream into total body water. It follows a three-compartment model of distribution, which is important for managing and removing the drug from the system.

Lithium is not metabolized in the body and is predominantly eliminated via the kidneys. Under normal conditions, about 80% of the filtered lithium is reabsorbed in the proximal tubule, with only 20% excreted in the urine. The renal clearance rate is between 10-40 mL/min, and the elimination half-life is 20 to 24 hours.

Clinical Features

Acute Lithium Overdose:

Acute overdose, particularly from lithium carbonate, typically leads to gastrointestinal symptoms, including nausea, vomiting, abdominal pain, and diarrhea. These symptoms may cause significant fluid and electrolyte loss, particularly if more than 25 g of lithium is ingested, although smaller doses may also cause gastrointestinal distress.

Acute overdose does not usually cause significant neurotoxicity unless renal function is impaired, allowing lithium to accumulate in tissues.

Chronic Lithium Toxicity:

Chronic toxicity often results from prolonged lithium therapy, especially when renal function is impaired due to underlying illnesses or drug interactions. Conditions such as renal failure, congestive heart failure, dehydration, and sodium depletion can all impair lithium excretion.

Drugs like NSAIDs, SSRIs, ACE inhibitors, and thiazide diuretics can exacerbate lithium toxicity by decreasing renal clearance.

Neurological symptoms are common in chronic toxicity and include tremors, hyperreflexia, ataxia, and agitation. Severe cases may progress to stupor, rigidity, hypotension, and life-threatening conditions like seizures and cardiovascular collapse.

Clinical Investigations

Key investigations for assessing lithium toxicity include:

Serum electrolytes, renal function tests, and a serum lithium concentration. Serial monitoring of lithium levels may be necessary for accurate management.

Therapeutic lithium concentrations typically range from 0.6 to 1.2 mEq/L. Toxicity can occur at levels above this, especially in older individuals. Levels of 1.5 to 2.5 mEq/L are associated with mild toxicity, 2.5 to 3.5 mEq/L with severe toxicity, and levels greater than 3.5 mEq/L are life-threatening.

In cases of acute overdose, lithium levels may not correlate with clinical symptoms as they do not directly reflect CNS concentrations. Serial monitoring can be useful to guide treatment decisions.

Treatment

Acute Lithium Overdose:

Most cases of acute overdose are managed with supportive care, including intravenous fluids (normal saline) to correct electrolyte imbalances and maintain adequate urine output.

Excessive hydration or forced diuresis does not enhance lithium elimination and should be avoided.

Activated charcoal is ineffective for lithium poisoning and should only be considered if there has been a significant co-ingestion.

Whole-bowel irrigation may be recommended for large overdoses of extended-release formulations.

Hemodialysis is rarely needed in cases of acute overdose with normal renal function but may be considered if renal failure or neurotoxicity develops.

Chronic Lithium Toxicity:

The diagnosis of chronic toxicity should be suspected in any patient on lithium therapy presenting with neurological symptoms.

Management focuses on supportive care, enhancing renal function, and correcting fluid and sodium imbalances with intravenous saline.

Lithium therapy and any contributing medications should be discontinued.

Hemodialysis may be considered in severe cases of chronic toxicity with life-threatening neurotoxicity. Although it is effective in removing lithium from the body, its effect on clinical outcomes is unclear.

Indications for hemodialysis include lithium levels greater than 4.0 mEq/L, severe neurotoxicity, and life-threatening arrhythmias. The goal is to lower lithium concentrations to below 1 mEq/L or achieve clinical improvement.

Disposition and Prognosis

Chronic Lithium Toxicity: Patients require hospitalization for monitoring and treatment of electrolyte imbalances, renal function, and lithium levels. Hemodialysis may be necessary for severe cases. Neurological recovery can be slow, and permanent deficits may occur, especially in cases of irreversible lithium-effectuated neurotoxicity (SILENT).

Acute Lithium Overdose: The prognosis is generally good with appropriate supportive care. Once lithium levels fall below 2 mEq/L and the patient is asymptomatic, they can often be discharged. However, close monitoring is required to ensure the resolution of symptoms.

Chapter 6
Paracetamol Poisoning

Key considerations

1. Paracetamol poisoning is one of the most prevalent toxicological emergencies seen in emergency departments across Australasia.

2. The decision to administer antidotal treatment after a single acute paracetamol ingestion should be made using the paracetamol treatment nomogram.

3. N-acetylcysteine (NAC) effectively prevents liver damage, but its protective effect diminishes as the time to treatment increases. In cases where patients present more than 8 hours post-ingestion, NAC should be started while awaiting serum paracetamol concentrations and liver function results.

4. The paracetamol treatment nomogram is not applicable for assessing the risk of hepatotoxicity from repeated supratherapeutic doses.

5. Paracetamol overdose should be considered in patients with suspected self-poisoning, particularly those presenting with altered mental status or unexplained liver dysfunction.

6. A modified-release formulation of paracetamol is available in Australia, which should be identified when taking the drug history.

7. Standard NAC dosing may not suffice to prevent hepatotoxicity in cases of massive paracetamol ingestion (>50 g or 0.5 to 1 g/kg). Consultation with a clinical toxicologist is advised.

8. If the timing of paracetamol ingestion is unclear or the history of exposure is unreliable, NAC should be started and continued until the

infusion is complete, or until the clinical scenario can be clarified and no biochemical evidence of liver toxicity is found.

Introduction

Paracetamol poisoning is a common occurrence in Australia and other Western countries. In the United States, over 100,000 paracetamol poisoning cases are reported annually to the American Association of Poison Control Centers. In the United Kingdom, paracetamol accounts for over 40% of poisonings presenting to emergency departments.

Pharmacokinetics and Pathophysiology

Paracetamol (also known as acetaminophen) is rapidly absorbed from the gastrointestinal tract, with peak plasma concentrations reached within 30 to 60 minutes following the ingestion of immediate-release tablet formulations, and less than 30 minutes for liquid forms. The bioavailability of paracetamol increases with dose size, ranging from 68% after 500 mg to 90% after 1 to 2 g orally. The time to peak plasma concentration can be delayed by co-ingestants that slow gastric emptying, such as opioids, antihistamines, and anticholinergic agents.

The volume of distribution is approximately 1 L/kg, with about 50% of paracetamol bound to plasma proteins. Paracetamol undergoes metabolism primarily in the liver, with small amounts eliminated through the kidneys. Metabolites are excreted in the urine, with less than 4% remaining unchanged.

Under normal dosing conditions, about 60% of paracetamol is conjugated with glucuronide, 35% with sulfate, and less than 5% is metabolized by the cytochrome P450 system, particularly the CYP2E1 enzyme. This results in the production of a reactive metabolite, N-acetyl-p-para-benzoquinoneimine (NAPQI).

NAPQI is conjugated with glutathione, forming non-toxic metabolites that are excreted in the urine.

In cases of overdose, the glucuronidation and sulfation pathways become saturated, and paracetamol is increasingly metabolized via the cytochrome P450 system. When glutathione stores are depleted by more than 70%, NAPQI accumulates in the liver, binding to hepatocytes and causing cell death, leading to hepatic necrosis, especially in the centrilobular regions of the liver.

Chronic alcohol consumption or malnutrition can enhance paracetamol's microsomal metabolism, while acute alcohol ingestion and 4-methylpyrazole inhibit this process. However, cimetidine does not reduce the excretion of paracetamol metabolites and has no proven role in preventing hepatotoxicity after paracetamol poisoning.

In Australia, a modified-release formulation of paracetamol (Panadol Osteo) has been available since 2002 for managing arthritis pain. This formulation releases paracetamol gradually to maintain therapeutic concentrations over 8 hours. However, it has been associated with delayed peak serum concentrations, which may be undetected if only a single serum test is conducted within 4 hours. In severe overdose cases, particularly with opioids or other agents that delay gastric emptying, the delayed absorption can result in prolonged elevated serum levels, necessitating longer treatment with NAC.

Clinical Features

In the early stages of paracetamol poisoning, symptoms are nonspecific and may include mild nausea, vomiting, and malaise, typically occurring within the first 24 hours. During this time, paracetamol is metabolized, and glutathione stores begin to deplete. In severe cases, slight elevations in liver enzymes may be observed as early as 16 hours after ingestion.

Stage 2 (24-48 hours) is marked by a resolution of initial symptoms but the onset of right upper quadrant pain, hepatic tenderness, and worsening liver function with increasing transaminases, bilirubin, and prothrombin time.

Stage 3 (72-96 hours) involves a further deterioration in liver function, with the development of jaundice, encephalopathy, and possible chemical hepatitis. Peak levels of liver enzymes typically occur around 72 hours post-ingestion. Stage 4 is characterized by either recovery, marked by a decrease in aminotransferase levels, or the progression to fulminant hepatic failure, which may result in renal failure due to hepatorenal syndrome or direct nephrotoxicity from NAPQI.

Massive overdose may also lead to mitochondrial dysfunction, manifesting as coma, lactic acidosis, hypothermia, and hyperglycemia.

Uncommon sequelae may include acute renal failure or pancreatitis.

Assessment of Risk for Hepatotoxicity

The likelihood of hepatotoxicity following paracetamol overdose is dose-dependent. For healthy adults, hepatotoxicity can occur with an ingestion of more than 200 mg/kg or 10 g, whichever is lower. In children under 6 years, toxicity can occur with doses exceeding 200 mg/kg. The risk may be higher in individuals with pre-existing liver conditions, severe malnutrition, or those using enzyme-inducing substances.

The paracetamol treatment nomogram is a valuable tool for assessing the risk of hepatotoxicity based on serum paracetamol concentration 4 hours after ingestion. It correlates serum levels with the risk of liver damage, with concentrations above 1000 μmol/L (150 mg/L) at 4 hours indicating a significant risk of hepatotoxicity. If serum concentrations are above 2000 μmol/L (300 mg/L) at 4 hours, the risk increases to 87%. The treatment line at 1000 μmol/L (150 mg/L) at 4 hours provides a margin of safety, as confirmed by large-scale studies in the United States.

Repeated supratherapeutic doses of paracetamol, particularly in individuals with liver risk factors, can also lead to hepatotoxicity. Cases of liver failure have been reported even with chronic use of as little as 4 g per day in patients with underlying conditions such as acute illness or decreased oral intake.

Antidotal Therapy with Acetylcysteine in Paracetamol Poisoning: A Case-Based Overview

Acetylcysteine (NAC) remains the primary antidotal therapy for preventing liver toxicity following paracetamol (acetaminophen) overdose, particularly in cases where serum alanine transaminase (ALT) or aspartate transaminase (AST) exceed 1000 IU/L. The therapeutic effects of NAC are attributed to its role as a precursor for glutathione, which is essential for neutralizing the toxic metabolite NAPQI (N-acetyl-p-benzoquinone imine). Additionally, NAC contributes to hepatic sulfation, further minimizing the conversion of paracetamol into harmful metabolites.

In Australia, NAC administration follows the 20-hour intravenous protocol outlined by Prescott, involving an initial dose of 150 mg/kg over 15 minutes, followed by 50 mg/kg over 4 hours, and 100 mg/kg over 16 hours. However, some centers have transitioned to a simpler two-bag regimen (200 mg/kg over 4 hours and 100 mg/kg over 16 hours), which has been associated with fewer and less severe adverse reactions while maintaining comparable hepatotoxicity outcomes.

Timing of NAC Administration: The need for NAC is determined by the timing of paracetamol ingestion. When administered within 8 hours of overdose, the risk of developing hepatotoxicity is minimal (1%–6%), regardless of whether the drug is given intravenously or orally. However, the risk of toxicity rises significantly when treatment is delayed. If NAC is administered 10–16 hours after ingestion, the incidence of hepatotoxicity increases to 40%, and up to 87% if treatment is delayed further (16–24 hours). Despite this, NAC continues to limit liver damage even in late-presenting patients. For massive ingestions (e.g., >50g), or cases where paracetamol concentrations remain elevated, extended NAC therapy beyond the standard 20-hour regimen may be necessary.

Adverse Reactions to NAC: The most common adverse reactions to intravenous NAC include non-IgE-mediated histamine release (e.g., urticaria, bronchospasm, hypotension), which typically occurs during or immediately after the initial loading dose, as well as gastrointestinal symptoms (nausea, vomiting) associated with the sulfhydryl groups in NAC. While these reactions are often mild and respond to adjusting the infusion rate or administering antihistamines, the incidence of non-IgE-mediated reactions can reach up to 20%. Evidence from a prospective study suggests a slight reduction in these reactions when NAC is infused over 1 hour instead of the standard 15 minutes, although this difference is not statistically significant.

A retrospective review of a two-bag regimen revealed a reduction in severe reactions, from 10% with the three-bag regimen to just 4% with the simplified approach. In cases of prior adverse reactions to NAC, rechallenging with NAC may still be appropriate after adjusting the infusion rate or providing supportive care.

Management Based on Ingestion Timing:

1. Acute Overdose (Within 8 hours of ingestion):

Gastrointestinal Decontamination: Activated charcoal (AC) is recommended if the patient is cooperative and presents within 2 hours of ingestion. AC administration can reduce the paracetamol concentration, potentially lowering the need for NAC therapy.

NAC Administration: NAC therapy should be initiated if the serum paracetamol concentration exceeds the threshold on the nomogram. Clinically stable patients treated within 8 hours do not require further blood tests if they remain asymptomatic and do not fall into high-risk categories.

2. Acute Overdose (8 to 24 hours post-ingestion):

Due to the increased risk of hepatotoxicity, NAC should be initiated promptly. Serum paracetamol levels and liver function tests (LFTs) should be obtained. If the serum paracetamol level is below toxic thresholds and LFTs are normal, NAC may be discontinued. Otherwise, a full 20-hour NAC course should be administered, with possible extension if liver enzymes rise during treatment.

3. Acute Overdose (More than 24 hours post-ingestion):

Patients presenting more than 24 hours after ingestion may still benefit from NAC, particularly if serum paracetamol levels are detectable and/or there is evidence of hepatic injury. NAC should be continued at a dose of 100 mg/kg every 12 hours until the patient shows improvement in liver function or requires a liver transplant.

4. Acute Overdose with Unknown Time of Ingestion:

For cases with an uncertain ingestion timeline (e.g., due to altered mental status or co-ingestants), NAC should be administered empirically to avoid delays in therapy. If serum paracetamol concentration and LFTs indicate a non-toxic overdose, NAC may be discontinued after the standard 20-hour infusion.

5. Staggered Acute Overdose:

In situations involving multiple paracetamol overdoses over a period of hours, a worst-case scenario is adopted by assuming the total ingested dose was consumed as a single dose at the earliest possible time. Treatment is then based on this assumption using the nomogram, with therapy initiated if the serum concentration exceeds the threshold.

6. Repeated Supratherapeutic Ingestion:

For patients who repeatedly ingest paracetamol in supratherapeutic doses, risk of hepatic injury increases if more than 200 mg/kg or 10 g are ingested in 24 hours. In these cases, a biochemical risk assessment is necessary. If serum paracetamol levels exceed 132 µmol/L and/or aminotransferases are elevated, NAC should be initiated, and LFTs reassessed after 8 hours.

7. Paracetamol-Induced Hepatic Failure:

Though rare, paracetamol-induced hepatic failure can occur, especially in patients presenting late. Risk factors include elevated INR, hypoglycemia, thrombocytopenia, and encephalopathy. Prolonged NAC therapy may be required in these cases, along with supportive care in a liver unit, and consultation with a liver transplantation team is advised.

8. Modified-Release Paracetamol Overdose:

Ingestions of extended-release formulations of paracetamol (e.g., Panadol Osteo) may lead to delayed peak serum concentrations and necessitate prolonged monitoring. NAC should be initiated if the ingested dose exceeds 200 mg/kg or 10 g, with serum paracetamol levels monitored every 4 hours. If concentrations remain high, NAC therapy should continue beyond 20 hours.

9. Liquid Paracetamol Ingestion in Children (<6 Years Old):

Children under 6 years who ingest >200 mg/kg of liquid paracetamol should have their serum paracetamol concentration measured 2 hours after ingestion. If levels exceed 1000 µmol/L, NAC treatment should begin, with a follow-up test at 4 hours.

Conclusion: The timely administration of NAC remains a cornerstone in the management of paracetamol overdose, particularly in preventing hepatotoxicity. The treatment approach is tailored based on the timing of ingestion, with increasing urgency for later presentations. Monitoring for adverse reactions is crucial, but these are generally manageable. Prolonged or adjusted NAC therapy may be necessary in severe cases, and consultation with clinical toxicologists is recommended for challenging cases involving massive ingestions or delayed presentations.

Chapter 7
Salicylate Poisoning

Key Considerations

1. The pharmacokinetics of salicylates become significantly altered following an overdose, complicating their metabolism and elimination.

2. Treatment decisions, including patient disposition, rely on clinical signs, biochemical results, and trends in serum salicylate levels.

3. The primary goal of treatment is to minimize both metabolic disturbances and central nervous system toxicity associated with overdose.

4. Urinary alkalinization is a proven method to enhance the elimination of salicylates after an overdose.

5. In severe salicylate toxicity, mechanical ventilation may worsen acidosis by interfering

with the patient's ability to generate high minute volumes due to salicylate-induced hyperpnea.

6. Chronic salicylate poisoning, which often affects the elderly, presents as a gradual onset of metabolic acidosis that may be mistakenly attributed to other medical conditions.

Introduction

Salicylate, commonly found in various pharmaceutical formulations and over-the-counter products like herbal remedies, cough treatments, and topical agents, is a well-known compound used primarily for its analgesic and anti-inflammatory properties. However, salicylate poisoning is rare in Australian emergency departments, largely because paracetamol is preferred for pain relief. When acute salicylate poisoning occurs, it manifests in a predictable, dose-dependent manner, with a range of symptoms and signs that emergency physicians are trained to manage.

Chronic salicylate toxicity, however, is more frequently seen in elderly patients with multiple coexisting conditions and may require interventions such as hemodialysis due to its serious morbidity and mortality. Children rarely ingest enough aspirin to experience toxicity, but even small amounts of topical products containing methyl salicylate (e.g., more than 5 mL) can be hazardous in children under 5 years old. Close attention should be paid to the units of measurement (standard or SI) when interpreting serum concentrations to avoid errors.

Pharmacology and Pathophysiology

Aspirin (acetylsalicylic acid, ASA) is absorbed in the acidic environment of the upper gastrointestinal tract, where it is quickly converted into salicylic acid. Therapeutic doses peak in the bloodstream within 2 hours, though absorption can be delayed in overdose cases due to pylorospasm or the formation of pharmacobezoars. Sustained-release or enteric-coated aspirin formulations may result in peak serum concentrations up to 24 hours after ingestion.

Salicylic acid has a pKa of 3.0 and exists primarily in its non-ionized form at physiological pH (7.4). It is highly protein-bound (85-90%) in the bloodstream at therapeutic doses, with a low apparent volume of distribution. In overdose situations, the saturation of plasma protein binding causes free salicylate levels to rise. As the pH of the body decreases, more salicylate exists in its unionized form, facilitating its movement into tissues such as the central nervous system (CNS), increasing its distribution and toxicity.

The liver and kidneys metabolize salicylic acid, with the metabolites excreted in the urine, along with small amounts of unchanged salicylate. At therapeutic levels, the half-life of salicylate is around 4 hours. However, once concentrations exceed the therapeutic range, metabolism becomes saturated, shifting from first-order to zero-order kinetics, which significantly prolongs elimination. Urinary excretion is influenced by urine pH: alkaline urine increases the ionization of salicylate, preventing reabsorption in the renal tubules, thus enhancing excretion. For instance, raising urine pH from 5.0 to 8.0 can increase salicylate excretion by up to 1,000 times.

Aspirin's therapeutic effects (analgesic, antipyretic, antiplatelet, and anti-inflammatory) result from its ability to irreversibly inhibit cyclooxygenase enzymes (COX-1 and COX-2), thereby blocking prostaglandin synthesis. Overdose, however, leads to toxic effects on the CNS, acid-base balance, cellular metabolism, coagulation, lungs, and gastrointestinal system. CNS effects include respiratory stimulation, resulting in primary respiratory alkalosis, along with symptoms such as tinnitus, deafness, and confusion. Severe poisoning can lead to coma, seizures, and cerebral edema, especially when systemic acidosis facilitates the passage of unionized salicylate into the brain.

Metabolically, salicylates uncouple oxidative phosphorylation and inhibit key enzymes in the Krebs cycle, leading to acidosis, hyperglycemia, hyperthermia, and metabolic disruptions. Increased oxygen consumption and CO_2 production are also observed. Additionally, salicylate toxicity can lead to dehydration from excessive fluid loss through hyperventilation, fever, and vomiting. Though platelet aggregation is inhibited, major hemorrhage is rare. Non-cardiogenic pulmonary edema is also a recognized complication of severe toxicity.

Clinical Features

The severity of toxicity following salicylate ingestion is directly related to the dose consumed (see Table 25.7.1). The most critical elements for assessing risk include the clinical presentation, acid-base disturbances, serum salicylate levels, and the reported dose.

Chronic salicylate poisoning often presents more subtly and may be difficult to diagnose.

Repeated aspirin use, especially in the context of viral illnesses or chronic pain, can lead to the accumulation of salicylate in the bloodstream, prolonging its elimination half-life. Symptoms may initially be nonspecific, resembling infections or inflammatory conditions, such as fever, dehydration, confusion, and hyperglycemia. The history of excessive aspirin use may be overlooked, and the clinical symptoms could be misattributed to other conditions such as sepsis, myocardial infarction, or diabetic ketoacidosis. A key indicator of chronic toxicity is unexplained metabolic acidosis, which should raise suspicion. Early diagnosis is crucial, as delayed recognition increases the risk of morbidity and mortality.

Clinical Investigations

Salicylate poisoning should be suspected in patients exhibiting signs of toxicity, particularly if respiratory alkalosis and metabolic acidosis are present. Initial tests should include serum electrolytes, blood glucose, creatinine, urea,

INR, paracetamol, and salicylate levels. Blood gas analysis (arterial or venous) is essential to assess the acid-base status, while urine pH should also be measured.

In mild poisoning, respiratory alkalosis may be observed due to the direct stimulation of the respiratory center, with concurrent hypokalemia. The urine pH may be initially alkaline due to hyperventilation. In cases of moderate-to-severe poisoning, a mixed acid-base disturbance of respiratory alkalosis and metabolic acidosis is common. Urine pH is often acidic, reflecting increased excretion of hydrogen ions. In severe cases, a metabolic acidosis with normal or decreasing serum pH may suggest progression to critical poisoning.

For effective monitoring, serial clinical observations, blood-gas measurements, and salicylate concentration testing should be used to track the ongoing absorption and assess treatment effectiveness.

Treatment

Initial management of salicylate poisoning includes securing intravenous access and obtaining blood samples for salicylate levels, electrolytes, and glucose. In moderate-to-severe cases, these tests should be repeated every 3 to 4 hours due to the erratic absorption of salicylate. Rehydration is crucial, particularly in patients who may be at higher risk (e.g., young children, elderly individuals, or those with cardiac conditions). Monitoring central venous pressure or arterial pressure may be necessary in severe cases, as well as urinary catheterization for hourly urine measurements.

Gastrointestinal decontamination with activated charcoal is recommended for all patients who present soon after ingestion, even if several hours have passed since the overdose, given the potential for delayed absorption. For large ingestions, particularly with sustained-release or enteric-coated aspirin formulations, whole-bowel irrigation with polyethylene glycol-electrolyte solutions may be considered. Repeated doses of activated charcoal may be useful if serial serum salicylate levels continue to rise, though it does not enhance salicylate elimination.

Treatment of pulmonary edema should involve continuous positive pressure ventilation, either via mask or endotracheal intubation. Salicylate toxicity often results in high minute ventilation and respiratory alkalosis, necessitating ventilation strategies that ensure adequate oxygenation and prevent respiratory acidosis. Seizures should be managed with benzodiazepines.

Urinary alkalinization is the primary method for enhancing salicylate elimination. This treatment can reduce the elimination half-life from 20 hours to about 5 hours. The goal is to raise the urine pH above 7.5, which increases the ionization of salicylate, trapping it in the renal tubules and preventing its reabsorption. Indications for urinary alkalinization include the presence of tinnitus, significant acid-base disturbances, or serum salicylate levels above 2.2 mmol/L (30 mg/dL). Urinary alkalinization should be initiated while awaiting test results in symptomatic patients.

To alkalinize the urine, an intravenous loading dose of sodium bicarbonate (0.5 to 1.0 mmol/kg) is given, followed by a continuous infusion of sodium bicarbonate (100–150 mmol in 1 L of 5% dextrose at 100-250 mL/hour, adjusted based on urine pH). Urine output should be maintained at 1-2 mL/kg/hour, and serum potassium levels should be carefully monitored, as hypokalemia can interfere with the alkalinization process. In the presence of systemic hypokalemia, potassium supplementation is necessary to avoid potassium depletion during treatment.

Urinary alkalinization in salicylate poisoning can be challenging. To manage the overdose effectively, serial measurements of serum electrolytes, salicylate concentrations, and urinary pH should be performed every 3 to 4 hours. The primary goals of therapy are to achieve a reduction in serum salicylate levels to the therapeutic range (1.1 to 2.2 mmol/L or 15 to 30 mg/dL), resolution of clinical toxicity signs, and normalization of the acid-base balance.

Extracorporeal removal of salicylates is rarely necessary but may be indicated under specific conditions, such as severe intoxication. The clinical indications for hemodialysis (HD) include worsening metabolic acidosis, organ dysfunction, or high serum salicylate concentrations (greater than 6.0 mmol/L or 100 mg/dL). Intermittent high-flow hemodialysis is preferred because it can quickly correct acid-base, fluid, and electrolyte imbalances while removing salicylates from the bloodstream. Although sustained low-efficiency hemodialysis (SLED) may be considered, its effectiveness in severe cases remains uncertain due to a lack of comprehensive data.

In critical cases of salicylate toxicity, endotracheal intubation and mechanical ventilation might be required, either due to the direct effects of the poisoning or from co-ingested substances. Prior to intubation, intravenous sodium bicarbonate (1 to 2 mmol/kg) may be administered. Hyperventilation is also necessary to maintain respiratory alkalosis, a condition that helps mitigate the effects of acidosis. In these severe cases, continued urinary alkalinization and hemodialysis are crucial for treating the associated metabolic acidosis.

Disposition decisions are complicated by the potential for delayed or erratic salicylate absorption. Therefore, patients need to be observed for at least 12 hours and undergo serial salicylate testing. Early measurements (less than 6 hours post-ingestion) may not accurately reflect peak salicylate concentrations, which often occur later. Patients showing no clinical signs of toxicity and with normal blood gas levels and decreasing salicylate concentrations (within the therapeutic range) can be cleared for discharge. However, those with signs of acid-base disturbances, organ dysfunction, or ongoing need for urinary alkalinization should be admitted to a high-dependency or intensive care unit. Severe cases requiring hemodialysis or with significant toxicity should be transferred to a tertiary care facility.

Indications for Hemodialysis in Salicylate Poisoning

Hemodialysis is recommended for patients with:

Persistent worsening metabolic acidosis despite treatment

Evidence of end-organ damage (e.g., cerebral edema, seizures, rhabdomyolysis)

Renal failure or fluid overload

Serum salicylate concentrations above 6.0 mmol/L (100 mg/dL) in acute poisoning or 4.0 mmol/L (60 mg/dL) in chronic cases

Controversies
The threshold for initiating urinary alkalinization is not universally agreed upon, with many toxicologists recommending its use for symptomatic patients to minimize hospitalization duration. Although there is limited controlled evidence supporting continuous veno-venous hemodialysis (CVVHD) for severe salicylate toxicity, newer high-flow dialysis techniques, such as SLED, have been shown to effectively remove significant amounts of salicylate and may be an alternative in cases where standard high-flow dialysis is not accessible.

Chapter 8
Antidiabetic Drugs

Key Considerations

1. Deliberate overdose of insulin or sulfonylureas can result in severe hypoglycemia, requiring prolonged observation and treatment over several days.

2. Octreotide effectively blocks insulin secretion in cases of sulfonylurea toxicity, offering a therapeutic option in managing such overdose.

3. Central venous access may be necessary for delivering concentrated glucose solutions following an insulin overdose.

4. Metformin, while useful for diabetes management, is associated with life-threatening lactic acidosis but typically does not cause hypoglycemia in cases of overdose.

Introduction

Diabetes mellitus (DM) is a persistent metabolic disorder characterized by an absolute (type 1) or relative (type 2) insulin deficiency. In Australia, over one million people are affected, with an additional 100,000 diagnoses annually. Indigenous and Māori populations experience some of the highest rates of type 2 diabetes globally. This significant health burden has led to widespread use of antidiabetic drugs, which are frequently misused, either by diabetics or non-diabetics in overdose scenarios.

The main classes of antidiabetic medications are insulin, sulphonylureas, and biguanides, all of which have been in use for over 50 years. Toxicity can result from intentional overdose or reduced drug clearance due to liver or kidney dysfunction. Recently, newer drugs for type 2 diabetes have emerged, including DPP-IV inhibitors, incretin mimetics, thiazolidinediones, alpha-glucosidase inhibitors, glinides, and SGLT2 inhibitors, although overdoses of these drugs generally do not cause severe toxicity.

Insulin

Pharmacology and Pathophysiology

Insulin is synthesized by the pancreas in the form of proinsulin, which is then cleaved to produce active insulin and C-peptide. Exogenous insulin, used in the management of both type 1 and type 2 diabetes, lacks C-peptide. Insulin is primarily eliminated through hepatic metabolism (60%) and renal clearance (40%). After an overdose, the pharmacokinetics may be altered, as the insulin injected subcutaneously or intramuscularly may form a depot, leading to a delayed and erratic release that can extend its action for several days.

Insulin promotes the intracellular transport of glucose, potassium, magnesium, and phosphate, and inhibits the breakdown of fat and protein. In overdose situations, the primary clinical concern is hypoglycemia, which can be prolonged and severe, especially in non-diabetic patients. Insulin toxicity can also lead to electrolyte imbalances, including hypokalemia, hypophosphatemia, and hypomagnesemia.

Clinical Features

The symptoms of insulin overdose are largely due to hypoglycemia. These include autonomic signs such as diaphoresis, tremors, nausea, palpitations, and tachycardia, as well as neuropsychiatric manifestations such as confusion, agitation, seizures, coma, and focal neurological deficits. Symptoms often appear within hours of insulin overdose, with patients frequently presenting in a comatose state. Severe, prolonged hypoglycemia can result in permanent neurological damage or even death.

Clinical Investigations

Monitoring blood glucose is critical in managing insulin overdose. Serial electrolyte measurements are essential, particularly for potassium levels, as hypokalemia may develop. Magnesium and phosphate levels should also be monitored. In cases where intentional overdose is suspected, insulin and C-peptide levels can help differentiate exogenous insulin administration from endogenous insulin production.

Treatment

The primary management of insulin overdose is supportive, with the mainstay of treatment being the administration of concentrated dextrose solutions to correct hypoglycemia. Initially, 50% dextrose should be used, followed by a continuous infusion of 10% dextrose at 100 mL/h. Frequent monitoring and adjustments to the dextrose infusion rate may be required, sometimes for several days. Central venous access is often necessary for administering concentrated glucose solutions. In addition, hypokalemia should be addressed with potassium supplementation, carefully monitored to avoid overcorrection.

Oral complex carbohydrates can complement intravenous glucose to stabilize blood sugar levels more physiologically. Close monitoring for hyponatremia and volume overload is also necessary, particularly in patients receiving large volumes of dextrose.

Patients should be observed for at least 8 hours following an overdose. Discharge is possible if the patient remains asymptomatic and euglycemic. Those requiring ongoing dextrose therapy should be admitted to an intensive care unit for continued monitoring. Gradual weaning off dextrose is recommended to avoid abrupt hypoglycemia. In non-diabetic patients, the weaning process may be slower due to a rebound insulin secretion stimulated by large dextrose infusions.

Sulphonylureas

Pharmacology and Pathophysiology

Sulphonylureas, such as glibenclamide, gliclazide, glimepiride, and glipizide, are commonly prescribed oral hypoglycemics. These drugs work by binding to potassium channels on pancreatic beta cells, leading to insulin release. The duration of action is typically 12-24 hours but can be significantly prolonged in overdose situations. These drugs are metabolized in the liver and excreted. Toxicity is more pronounced in patients with hepatic or renal dysfunction, where drug accumulation may occur.

Clinical Features

Sulfonylurea-induced hypoglycemia can occur after therapeutic use, unintentional administration, or deliberate overdose. Overdoses often result in profound and prolonged hypoglycemia. Symptoms are similar to those of insulin overdose and include confusion, seizures, and coma. Treatment is focused on correcting hypoglycemia with dextrose, though it may be more resistant to correction than insulin-induced hypoglycemia.

Treatment

Immediate correction of hypoglycemia with dextrose is essential, starting with a bolus of 50 mL of 50% dextrose, followed by a 10% dextrose infusion. In cases of sulfonylurea overdose, the hypoglycemia is often refractory to dextrose alone, and early administration of octreotide is indicated to manage persistent hypoglycemia. Activated charcoal can be used in cases where the overdose occurred within a few hours, though it should not delay dextrose administration. In elderly patients, who often have comorbidities, managing sulfonylurea-induced hypoglycemia can be complex, requiring careful monitoring and potential use of octreotide.

Octreotide

Octreotide, a synthetic analogue of somatostatin, inhibits insulin release from pancreatic beta cells by blocking calcium influx. It is considered the first-line treatment for sulfonylurea-induced hypoglycemia. Octreotide therapy should be initiated early and can reduce or eliminate the need for dextrose infusions. The recommended initial dose is 50 μg IV, followed by a continuous infusion of 25 μg/h. Alternatively, 100 μg can be administered subcutaneously or intramuscularly every 6 hours. Treatment should continue for at least 24 hours.

Octreotide is well tolerated, although side effects such as nausea and vomiting are occasionally reported.

Disposition

Patients who overdose on sulphonylureas should be admitted for observation and monitored for at least 8 hours after ingestion. If hypoglycemia persists or worsens, intensive care and continuous monitoring are required. Once the patient is stable and euglycemic for 6 hours after discontinuing dextrose therapy, they may be discharged. All cases of deliberate overdose require psychiatric evaluation once the medical crisis is resolved.

References

1. Diabetes Australia, Canberra ACT. Available at: http://www.diabetesaustralia.com.au. Accessed January 2018.

2. Samuels MH, Eckel RH. "Massive insulin overdose: In-depth analysis of free insulin levels and glucose requirements." Clinical Toxicology. 1989; 27:157–168.

3. Haskell RJ, Stapczynski JS. "Duration of hypoglycemia and intravenous glucose need following insulin overdose." Annals of Emergency Medicine. 1984; 13:505–511.

4. McLaughlin SA, Crandall CS, McKinney PE. "Octreotide as an antidote for sulfonylurea-induced hypoglycemia." Annals of Emergency Medicine. 2000; 36:133–138.

5. Glatstein M, Scolnik D, Bentur Y. "Use of octreotide in treating sulfonylurea poisoning." Clinical Toxicology. 2012; 50:795–804.

6. Wills BK, Bryant SM, Buckley P, Seo B. "Can metformin overdose lead to lactic acidosis?" American Journal of Emergency Medicine. 2010; 28:857–861.

7. Spiller HA, Weber JA, Winter ML. "Multicenter case series on pediatric metformin ingestion." Annals of Pharmacotherapy. 2000; 34:1385–1388.

8. Dell'Aglio DM, Perino LJ, Todino JD. "Metformin overdose resulting in a serum pH of 6.59: Survival without sequelae." Journal of Emergency Medicine. 2010; 39:77–80.

9. Calello DP, Liu KD, Wiegand TJ, et al. "Extracorporeal treatments for metformin poisoning: A systematic review and recommendations from the Extracorporeal Treatments in Poisoning Workgroup." Critical Care Medicine. 2015; 43(8):1716–1730.

10. Darracq MA, Toy JM, Mo C, Cantrell FL. "A retrospective review of isolated gliptin exposure cases reported to a state poison control center." Clinical Toxicology. 2015; 52(3):226–230.

11. Lovshin JA, Drucker DJ. "Incretin-based therapies for type 2 diabetes mellitus." Nature Reviews Endocrinology. 2009; 5:262–269.

12. Elling R, Spehl MS, Wohlfarth A, et al. "Prolonged hypoglycemia after suicidal ingestion of repaglinide with unexpected slow plasma elimination." Clinical Toxicology.

Chapter 9
Colchicine Poisoning

Key Considerations

1. Self-Poisoning Risk: All cases of deliberate self-poisoning with colchicine must be considered life-threatening.

2. Initial Presentation: Symptoms may initially be absent or limited to gastrointestinal (GI) symptoms.

3. Diagnosis: Consider colchicine poisoning in patients with gastrointestinal symptoms that progress to multi-organ failure, particularly bone marrow failure.

4. Management: Early recognition of the severity of poisoning, prompt gastrointestinal decontamination, and aggressive supportive care are critical.

Introduction

Colchicine, an alkaloid extracted from Colchicum autumnale (Autumn Crocus) and Gloriosa superba (Glory Lily), is commonly used for treating conditions like acute gout, familial Mediterranean fever, scleroderma, primary biliary cirrhosis, and recurrent pericarditis. While rare, colchicine poisoning is most often a result of intentional overdose or therapeutic errors, especially in elderly patients or those with pre-existing liver or kidney disease. Severe toxicity, although uncommon with therapeutic doses, can still occur, often due to prolonged drug use or underlying health issues. Poisoning can also stem from consuming various parts of the Colchicum autumnale or Gloriosa superba plants.

The risks of colchicine poisoning are often underestimated, and the condition may be misdiagnosed at the initial presentation, contributing to delayed treatment and high mortality.

Toxicokinetics

Colchicine is absorbed rapidly from the small intestine, with peak plasma levels occurring within 0.5 to 2 hours after ingestion. Its oral bioavailability ranges from 25% to 40%, as it undergoes significant first-pass metabolism in the liver. Highly lipid-soluble and 50% protein-bound, colchicine distributes rapidly throughout the body, with a volume of distribution of 2 L/kg, which can increase significantly in cases of toxicity. The drug is primarily metabolized by the liver via CYP3A4, with a small portion eliminated by the kidneys. In cases of renal or hepatic impairment, drug clearance is markedly reduced, and the risk of toxicity increases, especially with drugs that inhibit CYP3A4 or P-glycoprotein.

Pathophysiology

Colchicine exerts its toxic effects by binding to tubulin, preventing its polymerization into microtubules, essential components of the cell cytoskeleton. Microtubules are involved in various critical cellular processes, including cell division, intracellular transport, and motility. When colchicine disrupts microtubules, it causes cell dysfunction and mitotic arrest, particularly in the rapidly dividing cells of the gastrointestinal mucosa and bone marrow. As a result, colchicine toxicity impacts nearly every organ system, including the cardiovascular, respiratory, and neurological systems.

Clinical Features

Colchicine poisoning typically follows a three-phase progression:

Stage 1 (0-24 hours)

Symptoms: GI distress (nausea, vomiting, diarrhea, abdominal pain), hypotension, and leukocytosis.

This phase may also present with intravascular volume depletion, requiring attention to fluid status.

Stage 2 (24-72 hours)

Symptoms: Multi-organ failure, including respiratory distress, bone marrow suppression, cardiovascular collapse, disseminated intravascular coagulation (DIC), and metabolic disturbances such as hypomagnesemia, hypocalcemia, and metabolic acidosis.

Neurological symptoms may include delirium, seizures, and coma.

Cardiovascular instability, arrhythmias, and renal failure are common and often fatal.

Stage 3 (6-8 days)

Symptoms: Recovery phase characterized by resolution of organ dysfunction, rebound leukocytosis, and potential alopecia.

Bone marrow function recovers, and hair loss is typically reversible.

Differential Diagnosis: Diagnosing colchicine poisoning can be challenging, especially when the history of ingestion is unclear or the symptoms mimic those of gastroenteritis, sepsis, or an acute abdomen. Healthcare providers should consider colchicine toxicity in cases of progressive multi-organ dysfunction after GI symptoms, especially when bone marrow suppression is evident.

Clinical Investigations: Given the risk of multi-organ failure, baseline investigations should include:

Electrolytes, full blood count, coagulation profile

Renal and liver function tests

Creatine kinase, ECG, chest X-ray

Leukocytosis is often observed early in the course of poisoning. However, measuring colchicine levels in biological fluids is generally not helpful for clinical management.

Treatment

The cornerstone of colchicine poisoning management is early recognition, gastrointestinal decontamination, and aggressive supportive care.

Gastrointestinal Decontamination

Activated charcoal may be administered if the patient presents within a few hours of ingestion. This may reduce the severity of symptoms by preventing further absorption of the toxin. For patients in the second phase, aggressive supportive care is prioritized over decontamination.

Supportive Care

Focus on maintaining urine output with intravenous fluids, correcting electrolyte imbalances, and managing cardiac and respiratory support. Inotropic agents, mechanical ventilation, and dialysis are generally ineffective due to colchicine's high volume of distribution.

Potential Interventions

In some cases, multi-dose activated charcoal may be considered in patients with renal or hepatic impairment. Use of granulocyte colony-stimulating factor (G-CSF) for bone marrow suppression has been reported but remains unproven. Anti-colchicine Fab fragments may offer a potential therapeutic option but are not commercially available.

Disposition

All suspected cases of colchicine overdose should be admitted for at least 24 hours of monitoring. Asymptomatic patients without gastrointestinal distress may be safely discharged after this observation period. However, those presenting with symptoms require intensive care unit admission for close monitoring.

Prognosis

The mortality rate in colchicine poisoning is high and largely depends on the ingested dose and the timing of medical intervention. Early resuscitation and supportive care can significantly improve outcomes, particularly in those presenting early in the poisoning process. Patients who survive the second phase of toxicity can generally expect full recovery, although they may experience transient alopecia, which resolves over time.

Controversies

The use of G-CSF in colchicine-induced bone marrow suppression is debated. Some reports suggest a positive response, but further evidence is needed to confirm its therapeutic benefit.

The potential role of anti-colchicine Fab fragments in treating severe toxicity shows promise based on animal studies, but their use in human cases is still investigational.

References

1. Putterman C, Ben-Chetrit E, Caraco Y, Levy M. Colchicine toxicity: insights into clinical pharmacology, associated risk factors, clinical presentation, and therapeutic strategies. Semin Arthritis Rheum. 1991;21(3):143–155.

2. Finkelstein Y, Aks SE, Hutson JR, et al. Colchicine poisoning: exploring the hazardous

effects of an ancient therapeutic agent. Clin Toxicol. 2010;48(5):407–414.

3. Borisy GG, Taylor EW. Investigating colchicine's mode of action: interaction with cellular proteins via colchicine-3H binding. J Cell Biol. 1967;34(2):525–533.

4. Stapczynski JS, Rothstein RJ, Gaye WA, Niemann JT. Colchicine overdose: a case series and literature review. Ann Emerg Med. 1981;10(7):364–369.

5. Bismuth C, Gaultier M, Conso F. Bone marrow aplasia following acute colchicine toxicity: analysis of 20 cases. Nouv Presse Med. 1977;6(19):1625–1629.

6. Jarvie D, Park J, Stewart MJ. High-performance liquid chromatography for colchicine quantification in poisoning cases. Clin Toxicol. 1979;14(4):375–381.

7. Iosefina I, Lan J, Chin C, et al. Recovery following a massive colchicine overdose. Case Rep Nephrol Dial. 2012;2(1):20–24.

8. Stemmermann GN, Hayashi T. Reevaluating colchicine toxicity: pathological insights from three fatal cases. Hum Pathol. 1971;2(2):321–332.

9. Sauder P, Kopperschmidt J, Jaeger A, Mantz JM. Hemodynamic findings in eight patients with acute colchicine poisoning. Hum Toxicol. 1983;2(2):169–173.

10. Zawahir S, Gawarammana I, Dargan PI, et al. The role of activated charcoal in reducing colchicine release from Gloriosa superba in simulated gastrointestinal environments. Clin Toxicol. 2017;55(8):914–918.

11. Harris R, Marx G, Gillett M, et al. Managing colchicine-induced bone marrow suppression with granulocyte colony-stimulating factors. J Emerg Med. 2000;18(4):435–440.

12. Baud FJ, Sabouraud A, Vicaut E, et al. Colchicine-specific Fab fragments in the treatment of severe overdose: a brief review. N Engl J Med. 1995;332(10):642–645.

13. Eddleston M, Fabresse N, Thompson A, et al. Preventing lethal colchicine toxicity with anti-colchicine Fab fragments: findings from a porcine model. Clin Toxicol. 2018;1–9.

Chapter 10
Theophylline and Caffeine

Key Considerations

1. Methylxanthine toxicity is a serious condition that can result in life-threatening seizures and cardiac arrhythmias.

2. Predictors of severe toxicity include hypokalaemia, lactic acidosis, and elevated serum theophylline levels.

3. Early recognition of high-risk patients allows for timely intervention, including enhanced elimination techniques, to prevent severe complications.

Introduction

Theophylline, a methylxanthine derivative similar to caffeine, is occasionally implicated in overdoses presenting to the emergency department. While theophylline use has declined, cases of caffeine overdose have increased in parallel.

Therapeutic theophylline levels range from 10 to 20 mg/L. Toxicity may occur in adults ingesting more than 10 mg/kg in a single dose, often leading to serum concentrations exceeding this range.

Pharmacokinetics

Absorption:
Theophylline is highly bioavailable (~100%), with absorption rates influenced by its pharmaceutical formulation. Sustained-release forms, common in prescriptions, can delay peak absorption by up to 15 hours after overdose.

Distribution and Metabolism

Following absorption, theophylline is rapidly distributed and metabolized by the cytochrome P450 system into active and inactive metabolites. Its metabolism is variable and exhibits saturable kinetics, meaning small increases in dosage can lead to disproportionate rises in serum concentration at high levels. Approximately 10% of the drug is excreted unchanged in urine.

Elimination

Endogenous elimination slows significantly during severe intoxication, contributing to prolonged toxicity.

Pathophysiology

The exact mechanisms of theophylline toxicity are not fully understood. Hypotheses include:

1. Phosphodiesterase inhibition, leading to elevated intracellular cyclic adenosine monophosphate (cAMP).

2. Increased catecholamine activity.

3. Adenosine receptor antagonism.

4. Disruptions in intracellular calcium transport.

Clinical Features

Syndromes of Theophylline Toxicity

Acute Toxicity

Often results from deliberate overdose (e.g., suicide attempts) or accidental administration. Toxicity occurs at doses >10 mg/kg, with life-threatening complications expected at >50 mg/kg.

Chronic Toxicity

More common, often linked to prolonged supratherapeutic ingestion, drug interactions, or hepatic metabolism interference. Elderly individuals are at higher risk.

System-Specific Manifestations

1. Gastrointestinal:
Severe, refractory vomiting is common.

2. Cardiovascular:

Sinus tachycardia is a hallmark sign.

Severe intoxication may lead to arrhythmias such as atrial fibrillation and ventricular tachycardia, along with hypotension from β2-mediated vasodilation.

3. Central Nervous System (CNS):
Anxiety, insomnia, tachypnoea, and seizures (often refractory and associated with poor outcomes) are observed.

4. Metabolic Effects:

Includes hypokalaemia, lactic acidosis, and hyperglycaemia.

Hypokalaemia results from catecholamine-induced intracellular potassium shifts.

5. Musculoskeletal:
Muscle pain, rigidity, and myoclonus may occur.

Chronic vs. Acute Presentations:

Chronic toxicity often involves seizures and arrhythmias at lower serum concentrations than acute cases. Symptoms may manifest earlier when sustained-release formulations are involved.

Diagnostic Evaluation

Serum Theophylline Concentrations:

Acute toxicity: Mild effects at 20–40 mg/L, moderate at 40–80 mg/L, and severe at >80 mg/L. Levels >100 mg/L indicate high lethality risk.

Chronic toxicity: Significant effects can occur at concentrations as low as 20–30 mg/L, especially in patients over 60 years old.

Additional Investigations

Routine monitoring of electrolytes, liver function tests (LFTs), glucose, creatinine, and ECG is essential.

Management

Initial Supportive Care

Airway, breathing, circulation (ABC): Critical for managing life-threatening symptoms.

Hypotension: Responds to IV fluids; vasopressor infusions (e.g., noradrenaline) may be needed in refractory cases.

Arrhythmias: Managed with β-blockers (e.g., esmolol or metoprolol), though bronchospasm risk must be considered.

Seizures: Aggressively treated with benzodiazepines; refractory cases may require phenobarbital, propofol, or thiopentone.

Enhanced Elimination

Activated Charcoal: Useful post-overdose, even when presentation is delayed, provided vomiting is controlled.

Hemodialysis: Highly effective for theophylline clearance, especially in:

Acute poisoning with levels >100 mg/L.

Chronic poisoning >60 mg/L.

Severe complications (e.g., seizures, arrhythmias).

Alternatives include continuous venovenous hemofiltration (CVVH) or sustained low-efficiency dialysis (SLED) when standard hemodialysis is unavailable.

Disposition

All symptomatic patients require hospitalization.

Sustained-release formulations necessitate prolonged monitoring due to delayed toxicity onset.

Moderate-to-severe cases should be managed in monitored or intensive care settings.

Caffeine Toxicity

Caffeine toxicity mirrors that of theophylline, with symptoms such as palpitations, tremor, insomnia, and seizures. Severe overdoses may cause acute coronary syndromes. While laboratory confirmation of caffeine levels is rare, elevated theophylline (a caffeine metabolite) may serve as a surrogate marker.

Controversies

1. Charcoal Hemoperfusion:
Historically effective for theophylline removal but shows no clear clinical advantage over hemodialysis.

2. Continuous Renal Replacement Therapy (CRRT):
Useful in unstable patients but offers slower clearance rates compared to standard hemodialysis.

Chapter 11
Iron

Key Considerations

1. Acute iron poisoning poses a critical threat to life.

2. The severity of toxicity depends on the quantity of elemental iron ingested, not the weight of the iron salt.

3. Iron poisoning manifests both locally (gastrointestinal effects) and systemically.

4. Prompt gastrointestinal decontamination, including whole-bowel irrigation, is essential for managing high-risk cases.

5. Intravenous desferrioxamine serves as the cornerstone of treatment in severe cases and

should not be delayed for iron concentration results in critically ill patients.

6. While most patients recover, poor outcomes are associated with complications such as shock or coma.

7. Rare long-term complications include gastrointestinal scarring and obstruction.

8. The management approach for iron poisoning during pregnancy remains unchanged.

Introduction

Iron poisoning primarily affects preschool-aged children due to accidental ingestion. However, significant cases occur in adults, particularly in the context of intentional overdoses, including during pregnancy, given the widespread availability of iron supplements in obstetric care.

Iron is often perceived as a harmless dietary supplement, leading to unsafe storage and delayed medical intervention. Educational efforts, safer packaging, reduced dosages, and monitoring by poison control centers have led to a decline in iron toxicity over the past decade. Nevertheless, severe cases still arise.

Pathophysiology

Iron is crucial for red blood cell production, hemoglobin oxygenation, and various enzymatic functions. As the body cannot excrete iron directly, its levels are tightly regulated through the gastrointestinal (GI) tract. Upon absorption, iron binds reversibly to ferritin for storage or transferrin for transport to the bloodstream.

Iron is utilized in the bone marrow for hemoglobin synthesis or stored in the liver and spleen as ferritin or hemosiderin. The total iron-binding capacity (TIBC) reflects the maximum iron that transferrin can bind, typically exceeding serum iron levels by two to three times.

When iron demands are low, excess iron remains stored in intestinal cells. These cells eventually slough off, providing the primary mechanism for eliminating excess iron. However, free (unbound) iron, which is toxic to cellular processes, rarely occurs under normal conditions.

Local Effects

Iron salts exert a direct corrosive effect on the GI mucosa. In overdoses, this results in irritation, ulceration, bleeding, and, in severe cases, ischemia, infarction, or perforation. Fluid loss from GI damage can cause hypotension, shock, and metabolic acidosis.

Long-term effects of this corrosive action include scarring and strictures, potentially leading to gastrointestinal obstruction. The disrupted mucosa facilitates passive and enhanced iron absorption, worsening systemic toxicity.

Systemic Effects

Once the absorbed iron exceeds protein-binding capacity, free iron accumulates, leading to cellular dysfunction and death. Free iron localizes to mitochondria, generating free radicals that disrupt oxidative phosphorylation. Mitochondrial damage causes systemic manifestations such as cardiovascular collapse, metabolic acidosis, coagulopathy, and neurological symptoms, including encephalopathy.

Management

1. Gastrointestinal Decontamination:
Early decontamination is critical in severe poisoning cases. Whole-bowel irrigation is

particularly effective in preventing further iron absorption.

2. Chelation Therapy:
Intravenous desferrioxamine binds free iron, forming a complex excreted in the urine. This therapy should commence immediately in severe cases, without awaiting laboratory confirmation of elevated iron levels.

3. Supportive Care:
Monitoring and managing complications like shock, metabolic acidosis, or organ dysfunction are essential. Pregnant patients require identical treatment approaches, ensuring maternal and fetal well-being.

Prognosis

The majority of patients recover with timely intervention. However, the presence of shock or coma signifies a poor prognosis. Rare chronic complications include gastrointestinal scarring and obstruction.

Risk Assessment Based on Elemental Iron Dosage

Evaluating the severity of iron poisoning relies on the amount of elemental iron ingested per kilogram of body weight:

Asymptomatic: <20 mg/kg

Gastrointestinal (GI) symptoms only: 20–60 mg/kg

Risk of systemic toxicity: 60–120 mg/kg

Potentially lethal: >120 mg/kg

Accurate calculations must focus on elemental iron rather than the iron salt dosage. If the composition of the iron salt is unclear, a standard estimate of 105 mg of elemental iron per tablet should be used for assessment.

Pathophysiology of Iron Poisoning

Persisting metabolic acidosis after correcting hypovolemia and hypoperfusion indicates mitochondrial toxicity. Coagulopathy arises early due to impaired thrombin and clotting factor production, with later-stage effects attributed to hepatic dysfunction.

Prevention of Iron Poisoning

Iron poisoning remains a significant concern for young children, historically accounting for nearly one-third of toxicological deaths in the 1980s–1990s. The adoption of unit-dose packaging has significantly reduced accidental ingestions and related mortality. Ongoing public education further aids in minimizing incidences.

Clinical Features of Iron Poisoning

The progression of iron toxicity traditionally encompasses five stages, although the presentation and timeline vary among patients:

Stage 1 (0–6 hours): Gastrointestinal Toxicity

Common symptoms: vomiting, abdominal pain, diarrhea, and GI bleeding.

Severe cases may develop hypovolemic shock and metabolic acidosis due to fluid loss.

The absence of GI symptoms within six hours typically rules out significant poisoning.

Stage 2 (6–24 hours): Latent Phase

Known as the "quiescent phase," this stage reflects ongoing cellular toxicity despite the resolution of GI symptoms.

Patients recovering during this phase usually do not progress to systemic toxicity.

Stage 3 (6–48 hours): Systemic Toxicity

Characterized by shock, multiorgan failure, and metabolic acidosis.

Fatalities frequently occur during this stage due to combined effects of hypovolemia, vasodilation, and cardiac dysfunction.

Stage 4 (2–3 days): Hepatic Toxicity

Rare but severe, this phase features acute hepatic failure, including jaundice, hypoglycemia, and coagulopathy.

Stage 5 (2–6 weeks): Delayed Effects

Chronic complications, such as GI scarring, may cause gastric outlet obstruction or small bowel obstruction.

Investigative Tools for Diagnosis

Serum Iron Concentrations

Peak levels occur 2–6 hours post-ingestion but may be delayed in sustained-release formulations.

Serum iron concentrations above 90 μmol/L within 4–6 hours post-ingestion indicate high risk of systemic toxicity.

Serum iron levels alone may not correlate with clinical severity, as intracellular iron drives systemic effects.

Radiographic Imaging

Most iron preparations are radiopaque. Abdominal x-rays can confirm ingested tablets and guide decontamination efforts.

Negative x-rays do not exclude ingestion, particularly with liquid iron formulations or late presentations.

Other Diagnostic Markers

Anion-gap metabolic acidosis and elevated lactate levels signal systemic poisoning.

Tests such as liver and renal function panels, blood gases, and clotting profiles assist in monitoring severity.

Management of Iron Poisoning

General Approach

Management strategies depend on the ingested dose and symptom severity. Goals include supportive care, preventing systemic toxicity, and targeted treatments when necessary.

Supportive Care

Fluid replacement: Use isotonic fluids with boluses of 20 mL/kg as needed to maintain urine output.

For advanced toxicity: Inotropic support, blood transfusions, and correction of coagulopathy or acidosis may be required.

Gastrointestinal Decontamination

Whole-bowel irrigation (WBI): Recommended for ingestions >60 mg/kg of elemental iron with visible tablets on x-rays. Continue until rectal effluent is clear and no tablets are visible.

Gastric lavage: Reserved for life-threatening ingestions (>120 mg/kg) presenting within one hour.

Chelation Therapy

Desferrioxamine: The standard chelating agent binds ferric iron to form ferrioxamine, excreted in urine.

Indications

Systemic toxicity (shock, metabolic acidosis).

Serum iron >60 μmol/L with symptoms or >90 μmol/L post-ingestion even if asymptomatic.

Administer as a continuous IV infusion (15 mg/kg/hour).

Limit therapy to <24 hours to avoid pulmonary toxicity.

Adjust dose by 50% in severe renal failure.

Pregnancy Considerations

Pregnant patients with moderate-to-severe poisoning should receive desferrioxamine based on pre-pregnancy weight.

Enhanced Elimination

While hemodialysis and hemoperfusion are ineffective for iron removal, they may eliminate ferrioxamine complexes in renal failure patients.

Prognosis and Expert Consultation

Prompt and targeted intervention improves outcomes in iron poisoning.

Engage toxicologists for guidance on desferrioxamine use or in complex cases, including massive ingestions or refractory toxicity.

References

1. Bender PR, et al. "Cardiac Arrhythmias During Theophylline Toxicity." Chest, 1991.

2. Hall KW, et al. "Metabolic Abnormalities Associated with Theophylline Overdose." Ann Intern Med, 1984.

3. Shannon M, et al. "Life-Threatening Events After Theophylline Overdose." Arch Intern Med, 1999.

4. Gunja N, et al. "Energy Drinks: Health Risks and Toxicity." Med J Aust, 2012.

5. Ghannoum M, et al. "Extracorporeal Treatment for Theophylline Poisoning." Clin Toxicol, 2015.

Chapter 12
Drugs of Abuse

Key Considerations

1. Clinical Diagnosis: Diagnosing intoxication due to drugs of abuse is primarily clinical. Supportive care plays a critical role in optimizing patient outcomes.

2. Opioid Overdose: Contributing factors to opioid-related fatalities include co-ingestion of central nervous system (CNS) depressants, reduced tolerance, high drug purity, and hesitation to seek medical help. Naloxone is an essential intervention for airway and ventilation support in opioid overdoses.

3. Management of Amphetamine Toxicity: Benzodiazepines are pivotal in managing CNS and cardiovascular symptoms of amphetamine intoxication. Hyperthermia, reduced

consciousness, neurological signs, or chest pain signify life-threatening complications requiring immediate intervention.

4. Cocaine Toxicity: Cocaine use can lead to severe cardiac and non-cardiac toxicities, which may be fatal. Toxicity often mimics amphetamines but tends to have a shorter duration. Hyperthermia, seizures, chest pain, and arrhythmias demand prompt investigation and treatment.

5. Gamma-Hydroxybutyric Acid (GHB): This sedative-hypnotic drug causes CNS depression and is managed primarily with supportive care.

6. Synthetic Psychoactive Substances: These drugs exhibit varied effects due to constant structural modifications, making their impact unpredictable.

7. Prescription Drug Misuse: The illicit use of prescribed medications, particularly among older adults, is an escalating issue.

8. Emergency Department (ED) Intervention: Presentations to the ED following overdose offer opportunities for patient education and referrals for long-term rehabilitation.

Introduction

Illicit drug use accounts for 1.8% of disease burden and injury in Australia. In 2016, nearly 43% of Australians aged over 14 reported having used illicit drugs, with 15.6% indicating recent use within the past year. Commonly used substances include cannabis (10.4%), prescription and over-the-counter analgesics (3.6%), cocaine (2.5%), ecstasy (2.2%), and methamphetamine (1.4%).

While most users are adults aged 20 to 29, the average age of illicit drug users is rising. Adults over 50 now represent over 20% of users. Drug-related incidents affect 9% of the population annually.

Pharmaceutical Misuse

Pharmaceutical misuse involves the non-medical use of prescription or over-the-counter medications, exceeding prescribed dosages, or using them to achieve euphoric effects. Opioids, such as codeine and oxycodone, are the most commonly misused drugs. Efforts to restrict over-the-counter availability of codeine aim to curb misuse.

Risks and Complications

The assessment of drug misuse must consider:

Primary Toxic Effects: Resulting directly from the drug.

Complications of Use: Injection-related risks such as cellulitis, thrombophlebitis, and infections (e.g., endocarditis, bloodborne viruses).

Opportunity for Intervention: Emergency department visits serve as a critical point for education, counseling, and rehabilitation referrals.

Amphetamines

Pharmacology and Pathophysiology

Amphetamines, structurally similar to adrenaline, include derivatives such as methamphetamine, MDMA, and MDA. They can be ingested, smoked, insufflated, or injected, with peak serum levels occurring within 3 hours. These drugs enhance catecholamine release and inhibit reuptake, leading to intense CNS stimulation and sympathomimetic effects.

Clinical Features

Symptoms of amphetamine intoxication include:

Central Nervous System (CNS): Euphoria, agitation, psychosis, paranoia, hallucinations.

Peripheral: Tachycardia, hyperthermia, mydriasis, and diaphoresis.
Severe complications include myocardial infarction, rhabdomyolysis, intracranial hemorrhage, and renal failure. Chronic abuse may result in necrotizing vasculitis, renal impairment, and cardiovascular complications.

Management

Initial Stabilization: Focus on resuscitation and minimizing sensory stimuli.

Hyperthermia: Aggressive cooling measures, sedation with benzodiazepines, and, if necessary, paralysis with intubation.

Seizures: Benzodiazepines are first-line treatments. Barbiturates or general anesthesia may be required for refractory seizures.

Hyponatremia: Requires rapid sodium correction in cases linked to MDMA use.

Patients with mild symptoms may be discharged following observation, while those with persistent issues or severe toxicity may require hospitalization.

Cocaine

Pharmacology and Pathophysiology

Cocaine is derived from coca leaves and may be consumed in various forms, including hydrochloride (powder), freebase, or "crack" cocaine. It acts as a CNS stimulant by enhancing noradrenaline, dopamine, and serotonin levels while inhibiting their reuptake.

Clinical Manifestations

Cocaine use leads to CNS excitation, with symptoms such as agitation, seizures, and coma. Peripheral effects include tachycardia, hypertension, vasoconstriction, and hyperpyrexia. Severe complications include myocardial infarction, arrhythmias, and intracranial hemorrhage.

Management

Supportive Care: Manage seizures and hyperthermia aggressively.

Arrhythmias: Address underlying causes such as electrolyte imbalances and administer sodium bicarbonate if indicated.

Observation: Patients with mild intoxication may be monitored and discharged once stable, while those with severe symptoms require hospitalization.

Emerging Psychoactive Substances (EPS)

Introduction and Epidemiology

Emerging psychoactive substances (EPS), colloquially referred to as "legal highs," are synthetic compounds designed to mimic the effects of illicit drugs such as cannabis, MDMA, and hallucinogens. These substances are commonly obtained from online sources or specialty shops. In 2016, 2.8% of individuals aged 14 years and older reported lifetime use of synthetic cannabinoids, while 1% had experimented with other EPS.

The market for these substances is diverse, with inconsistent product compositions that often include unlisted illegal substances and caffeine. Constant development of new chemical analogues makes their clinical effects unpredictable and regulatory control challenging. EPS effects frequently resemble those of traditional illicit drugs. Below, the most common classes of EPS are reviewed.

Cathinones

Pharmacology and Pathophysiology

Cathinones, beta-ketone analogues of amphetamines, originate from the Catha plant (khat). Traditional khat chewing induces sympathomimetic effects. Synthetic analogues such as mephedrone, methcathinone, methylone, and MDPV ("bath salts") act by inhibiting monoamine reuptake. Typically ingested, insufflated, or injected, their effects begin within 15–45 minutes and last 2–7 hours.

Clinical Features

Cathinones produce heightened energy, reportedly more potent and enduring than cocaine. However, 20% of users experience adverse effects, including palpitations, gastrointestinal upset, and mental disturbances. Severe agitation, sympathomimetic toxidrome (chest pain, diaphoresis, tachycardia, and hypertension), psychosis, hallucinations, renal and liver dysfunction, rhabdomyolysis, hyponatremia, seizures, and death have also been documented.

Piperazines

Pharmacology and Pathophysiology

Benzylpiperazine (BZP) and trifluoromethylphenylpiperazine (TFMPP) are common piperazines. BZP acts as a dopamine reuptake inhibitor, enhancing catecholamine release and stimulating peripheral alpha-2 receptors. TFMPP is a serotonin agonist, particularly at 5-HT1 and 5-HT2 receptors. Metabolism through cytochrome P450 can lead to drug interactions.

Clinical Features

BZP and TFMPP are often combined to replicate MDMA's effects. Lower doses cause stimulant effects, while higher doses induce hallucinations. Symptoms include tachycardia, hypertension, agitation, confusion, gastrointestinal distress, hyperthermia, seizures, and psychosis. Some effects may persist for days, including lethargy, anxiety, and paranoia.

Synthetic Cannabinoid Receptor Agonists

Pharmacology and Pathophysiology

Synthetic cannabinoids, such as "spice" or "k2," activate CB1 and CB2 receptors with greater affinity than THC. These agents, often smoked in herbal mixtures, can also affect NMDA receptors. Overactivation of cannabinoid pathways results in sympathomimetic and hallucinogenic effects.

Clinical Features

Mild effects include tachycardia, diaphoresis, nausea, and agitation. Severe outcomes, such as myocardial ischemia, acute kidney injury, rhabdomyolysis, seizures, psychosis, and even death, are increasingly reported.

NBOMe

Pharmacology and Pathophysiology

N-methoxybenzyl (NBOMe) compounds, derivatives of phenylethylamine, mimic LSD. Their high affinity for serotonin (5-HT2A) and alpha-adrenergic receptors leads to potent hallucinogenic effects. These substances can be administered sublingually, nasally, or orally.

Clinical Features

Symptoms include tachycardia, agitation, hallucinations, hypertension, and confusion. Severe agitation may lead to self-injury or trauma. Serotonergic and sympathomimetic effects, such as hyperthermia and rhabdomyolysis, can result in kidney failure or death.

Clinical Investigations and Management

Diagnosis

EPS intoxication is primarily diagnosed clinically, as routine bedside drug tests often fail to detect these substances.

Treatment

Management is symptomatic and supportive. No specific antidotes are available. First-line treatment for agitation, seizures, and psychosis is intravenous benzodiazepines. Hyperthermia requires aggressive cooling measures and sedation. Hyponatremia should be corrected using established protocols.

Special Considerations: Opiates and Body Packers

Opiate Intoxication

Opiates, derived from Papaver , remain a significant cause of drug-related deaths.

Withdrawal symptoms—anxiety, nausea, diarrhea, and mydriasis—typically peak at two days and resolve within five days. Management includes hydration, symptom control, and referrals for addiction treatment.

Body Packers/Stuffers

Body-packers ingest large quantities of drugs for smuggling, while body-stuffers hastily conceal smaller amounts to evade authorities. Imaging modalities, such as non-contrast CT scans, are critical for diagnosis, with sensitivity nearing 100%. Treatment varies based on symptoms, ranging from conservative observation to surgical intervention in cases of bowel obstruction or toxicity.

Controversies

Optimal sedation regimens for stimulant intoxication.

Management of gamma-hydroxybutyrate (GHB) intoxication.

Best practices for handling EPS toxicity and gastrointestinal decontamination in body packers.

Chapter 13
Cyanide

Key Considerations

1. Cyanide is a highly lethal metabolic toxin requiring immediate recognition and intervention.

2. Toxicity manifests rapidly with effects on the central nervous system, respiratory system, cardiovascular system, and severe metabolic acidosis.

3. Elevated serum lactate levels are a reliable marker for cyanide exposure.

4. Immediate treatment with high-flow oxygen and appropriate antidotes is critical for survival, with several therapeutic options available.

5. Cyanide poisoning from smoke inhalation is frequently underdiagnosed and may be complicated by concurrent carboxyhemoglobinemia and methemoglobinemia, necessitating comprehensive management strategies.

Overview

Cyanide is a potent metabolic toxin associated with high fatality rates. Toxicity arises rapidly, impacting the central nervous, respiratory, and cardiovascular systems, often accompanied by severe metabolic acidosis. Elevated serum lactate levels strongly correlate with cyanide exposure. Immediate intervention with high-flow oxygen and antidotes can be life-saving, with several therapeutic options available. However, cyanide toxicity is frequently underdiagnosed in cases of smoke inhalation, where coexistence with carboxyhemoglobinemia or methemoglobinemia complicates management.

Introduction and Epidemiology

Cyanide encompasses any compound containing the cyano (CN) group and is used extensively in industries such as metal extraction (e.g., gold recovery), metal hardening, and the production of pesticides. Hydrogen cyanide (HCN), a highly toxic organic salt, exists in liquid or gaseous forms and has a characteristic bitter almond odor. However, 20–40% of individuals lack the genetic ability to detect this smell. Cyanide gas production in structural fires is well-documented, with toxic blood cyanide levels (>40 μmol/L) reported in most fire-related fatalities.

In cases involving severe burns, elevated lactate levels or carboxyhemoglobin levels >10% warrant consideration of cyanide antidotes. While blood cyanide concentrations can confirm exposure, the test's limited availability and delayed results necessitate clinical diagnosis. Lethal cyanide doses include ingestion of 200 mg or inhalation of HCN gas for approximately three minutes.

Historically, cyanide has been utilized in acts of mass homicide (e.g., Zyklon B during World War II), suicides, and is considered a potential chemical weapon due to its availability and capability to cause mass casualties. Cyanide can be dispersed as a gas or contaminant in water and food supplies, posing significant threats to public safety.

Toxicokinetics and Pathophysiology

Cyanide enters cells via rapid diffusion, with a half-life of 2–3 hours. Its primary mechanism involves binding to the ferric ion (Fe^{3+}) in cytochrome oxidase, inhibiting oxidative phosphorylation, halting ATP synthesis, and leading to lactic acid buildup. This disruption in cellular respiration results in metabolic acidosis and significant hydrogen ion accumulation. Additionally, cyanide affects neurotransmitter release in both the central and peripheral nervous systems.

The body detoxifies cyanide by converting it to thiocyanate (SCN) via enzymatic processes involving rhodanese and 3-mercaptopyruvate sulfurtransferase. However, the availability of these enzymes limits detoxification rates, emphasizing the importance of timely intervention.

Clinical Features

Acute cyanide poisoning presents rapidly, with symptoms ranging from mild to life-threatening. Symptom severity varies based on exposure route:

Neurological symptoms: Headache, dizziness, anxiety, disorientation, seizures, lethargy, and coma.

Respiratory effects: Initial hyperventilation progresses to respiratory depression due to central nervous system (CNS) impairment.

Cardiovascular effects: Hypertension followed by hypotension, tachycardia evolving into bradycardia, arrhythmias, and eventual cardiovascular collapse.

Skin findings, such as bright red discoloration due to impaired oxygen utilization, may not always be evident in severe cases.

Clinical Investigations

Timely diagnosis is crucial, but rapid cyanide assays are generally unavailable. Clinical diagnosis relies on findings such as elevated plasma lactate levels (>10 mmol/L), which strongly correlate with toxic blood cyanide levels (>40 µmol/L). Arterial blood gas analysis typically reveals metabolic acidosis.

Cyanide is concentrated in erythrocytes, and whole-blood cyanide levels guide toxicity assessment:

20 μmol/L: Symptomatic exposure

40 μmol/L: Toxicity

100 μmol/L: Potentially lethal

Advanced diagnostic tools, including environmental detectors, can aid prehospital assessment, especially for first responders.

Management and Treatment

Resuscitation

Immediate support of airway, breathing, and circulation is paramount. Administer 100% oxygen and ensure removal from enclosed spaces with high cyanide concentrations.

Rescuers must utilize protective gear to avoid exposure.

Decontamination

Skin and ocular exposures require thorough flushing with water or saline. Contaminated clothing should be removed and secured. Ingestion cases may benefit from activated charcoal, provided the airway is secure.

Antidotal Therapy

Empirical antidote administration is recommended when cyanide poisoning is strongly suspected, particularly in smoke inhalation victims with elevated lactate levels. Common antidotes include:

1. Hydroxocobalamin: A preferred first-line agent, it binds cyanide to form cyanocobalamin, excreted via urine.

2. Sodium Thiosulfate: Promotes conversion of cyanide to thiocyanate.

3. Sodium Nitrite: Induces methemoglobin formation, which competes for cyanide binding.

Antidote selection depends on patient condition, exposure scenario, and potential coexisting toxicities such as carboxyhemoglobinemia.

Supportive Care

Monitor cardiovascular and neurological status continuously. Treat seizures, hypotension, or arrhythmias as per advanced life support protocols.

Cyanide Antidotes: Simplified Overview

Cyanide poisoning is a medical emergency requiring immediate treatment with specific antidotes. These antidotes act through distinct mechanisms to detoxify cyanide and mitigate its toxic effects.

Hydroxocobalamin (Cyanokit)

Hydroxocobalamin is a first-line antidote recommended for severe cyanide poisoning. It binds cyanide directly to form cyanocobalamin, which is excreted via the kidneys. The standard dose is 5 grams administered intravenously over 15 minutes. In cases of severe poisoning, higher doses may be necessary. Clinical studies suggest it is safe and effective, even at elevated cyanide concentrations. Common side effects include temporary skin and urine discoloration, mild hypertension, headache, and bradycardia.

Sodium Thiosulfate

Sodium thiosulfate enhances the body's natural detoxification by promoting the conversion of cyanide to thiocyanate, a less toxic compound excreted in the urine. A typical dose is 12.5 grams administered intravenously over 10 minutes, which can be repeated if necessary. Side effects are generally mild, with nausea, vomiting, and headaches being the most common.

Nitrites

Nitrites, such as sodium nitrite and amyl nitrite, work by inducing methemoglobinemia. Methemoglobin binds cyanide, diverting it from interfering with cellular respiration. Sodium nitrite is administered as 300 mg intravenously over 5–20 minutes, while amyl nitrite is delivered via inhalation. Although effective, nitrites reduce the blood's oxygen-carrying capacity and may cause hypotension and vasodilation, making them less suitable for patients with co-existing carbon monoxide poisoning.

Dicobalt Edetate

Dicobalt edetate binds cyanide directly to form cobalt cyanide complexes. It is reserved for confirmed severe cyanide poisoning when safer alternatives are unavailable. The recommended dose is 300 mg intravenously over one minute. However, it carries significant risks, including anaphylaxis, hypotension, and cardiac arrhythmias, especially in individuals without cyanide poisoning.

Clinical Use and Recommendations

Hydroxocobalamin is the most widely recommended antidote due to its safety and efficacy profile. Sodium thiosulfate is also commonly used, particularly when other options are unavailable. While nitrites and dicobalt edetate remain viable alternatives, their side effects require careful patient selection. Early and aggressive supportive care, such as oxygen therapy and fluid resuscitation, is critical for improving outcomes. For all suspected cyanide poisoning cases, consultation with a toxicologist is strongly advised.

Controversies

The effectiveness of antidotes is primarily supported by animal studies and case reports, with limited data from human clinical trials. Hydroxocobalamin has shown consistent efficacy and is increasingly recognized as the preferred treatment, particularly in mass casualty scenarios involving cyanide exposure.

Chapter 14
Hydrofluoric Acid

Key Considerations

1. Unrecognized Hazard: Hydrofluoric acid (HF) is often unrecognized in household cleaning products, posing a risk to both patients and medical professionals.

2. Delayed Symptoms: Topical HF exposure may initially present with minimal physical signs but can cause severe pain disproportionate to the observed injury.

3. Immediate Decontamination: Irrigate skin immediately and thoroughly in cases of dermal exposure.

4. Escalation of Treatment: Persistent pain after dermal exposure requires escalation from topical calcium to more invasive methods, such as local

infiltration, intravenous, or intra-arterial calcium therapy.

5. Systemic Toxicity Risks: Exposure to high concentrations, large surface areas, or inhalation/ingestion can lead to systemic toxicity, including severe electrolyte imbalances, cardiac arrhythmias, and metabolic acidosis.

6. Electrolyte Imbalances: Common systemic manifestations include hypocalcemia, hypomagnesemia, hyperkalemia, and related complications.

Introduction

Hydrofluoric acid (HF) is a moderately corrosive inorganic compound, extensively utilized in industrial applications for etching glass, metals, and silicon, with concentrations typically ranging from 50% to 100%. Lower concentrations (<10%) are common in domestic cleaning agents such as rust removers and car wheel cleaners. Accidental exposure predominantly occurs via the skin, often due to compromised gloves in industrial settings or unprotected handling of domestic products. Inhalation and ingestion, although less common, pose significant risks in industrial and accidental contexts.

Pathophysiology

HF has a weak acidic nature (pKa = 3.8), resulting in limited immediate corrosive effects. Lower concentrations (<20%) allow the acid to penetrate deeper tissues without causing immediate pain, while higher concentrations (>50%) can induce immediate burning sensations. Tissue damage is primarily caused by fluoride ions, which bind divalent cations like calcium and magnesium, leading to hypocalcemia, hypomagnesemia, and coagulopathy. These interactions disrupt enzymatic processes and cellular respiration, impair Na+/K+ ATPase activity, and cause potassium leakage, culminating in hyperkalemia.

Unlike typical acid burns, HF exposure results in liquefactive necrosis, allowing deeper tissue penetration and significant injury.

Clinical Features

HF exposure is generally recognized in industrial settings, often accompanied by initial decontamination and relevant material safety data. However, domestic exposures may present diagnostic challenges due to delayed symptom onset, particularly with lower-concentration products.

Pain: The hallmark of HF exposure is severe pain disproportionate to physical signs. It often progresses from a tingling sensation to intense, throbbing pain.

Skin Manifestations: Early erythema and edema may evolve into blanching and a silvery-gray appearance, followed by vesiculation and necrosis if untreated.

Systemic Toxicity: Large surface area exposure (>5% BSA), high-concentration solutions (>20%), or inhalation/ingestion increases the risk of systemic effects, including electrolyte disturbances, metabolic acidosis, and cardiac arrhythmias.

Clinical Investigations

For minor dermal exposures involving less than 5% of BSA, investigations are usually unnecessary. However, significant exposure warrants serum electrolyte assessments (calcium, magnesium, potassium), coagulation studies, ECG monitoring, and chest imaging if respiratory symptoms are present.

Treatment

Initial Management

Immediate and thorough irrigation with water is crucial. Although alternative agents have been studied, evidence suggests no superiority over water in preventing systemic toxicity.

Topical calcium gluconate (2.5%-10%) should be applied promptly to neutralize fluoride ions.

Escalation of Therapy
If pain persists, escalation to localized or systemic calcium administration is required:

Local Injection: Direct infiltration of 10% calcium gluconate into affected tissues is effective but may be limited by anatomical constraints, particularly in digits.

Regional Infusion: In cases of limited injectable volume, regional intravenous infusion (e.g., Bier block) or intra-arterial infusion delivers calcium directly to affected tissues.

End Point: Pain relief is the clinical marker for effective treatment. Persistent pain may indicate irreversible tissue damage rather than ongoing fluoride ion activity.

Additional Considerations

Ocular Exposure: Requires immediate saline irrigation, with calcium gluconate solutions potentially added to irrigation fluid, though evidence of benefit is inconclusive.

Ingestion: Requires prompt gastrointestinal decontamination to minimize systemic absorption.

Prognosis and Complications

Delayed or inadequate treatment may lead to severe tissue destruction, systemic fluoride poisoning, and potentially fatal complications such as cardiac arrhythmias. Comprehensive and timely management can significantly mitigate morbidity and mortality associated with HF exposure.

References

1. Salzman, M., & O'Malley, R. N. (2007). Recent advances in the assessment and management of caustic exposures. Emergency Medicine Clinics of North America, 25, 459-476.

2. Burd, A. (2004). Revisiting hydrofluoric acid injuries. Burns, 30, 720-722.

3. Dunser, M. W., Ohlbauer, M., Rieder, J., et al. (2004). Critical care of significant hydrofluoric acid burns: A case report, literature review, and therapeutic recommendations. Burns, 30, 391-398.

4. Chan, B. S., & Duggin, G. G. (1997). Survival following substantial hydrofluoric acid

ingestion. Journal of Toxicology: Clinical Toxicology, 35, 307-309.

5. Graudins, A., Burns, M. J., & Aaron, C. K. (1997). Regional intravenous calcium gluconate infusion for hydrofluoric acid burns to the upper limbs. Annals of Emergency Medicine, 30, 604-607.

6. Caravati, E. M. (1988). Acute exposures to hydrofluoric acid. American Journal of Emergency Medicine, 6, 143-150.

7. Cummings, C. C., & McIvor, M. E. (1988). Fluoride-induced hyperkalemia: The role of calcium-dependent potassium channels. American Journal of Emergency Medicine, 6, 1.

8. Vance, M. V., Curry, S. C., Kunkel, D. B., et al. (1986). Treatment of hydrofluoric acid burns to the digits with intra-arterial calcium infusion. Annals of Emergency Medicine, 15, 890-896.

9. Hulten, P., Hojer, J., Ludwigs, U., et al. (2004). A comparison of Hexafluorine and standard decontamination in reducing systemic toxicity following dermal exposure to hydrofluoric acid. Journal of Toxicology: Clinical Toxicology, 42, 355-361.

10. Lin, T. M., Tsai, C. C., Lin, S. D., et al. (2000). Continuous intra-arterial calcium infusion for treating hydrofluoric acid burns. Journal of Occupational and Environmental Medicine, 42, 892-897.

Chapter 15
Pesticides - Detailed Overview

Key Considerations

1. Acute pesticide poisoning remains a significant global health concern, particularly in the Asia-Pacific region, with a notable contribution to morbidity and mortality rates.

2. Current pesticide toxicity classification systems are flawed. Even pesticides categorized as 'slightly hazardous' may exhibit severe toxicity. Moderate-to-highly toxic pesticides have a case-fatality rate ranging from 5% to 70%, especially in cases of self-poisoning.

3. The toxicity of pesticides is not solely determined by the active ingredient; co-formulants, such as solvents, surfactants, and salts, can exacerbate poisoning, leading to more

severe outcomes. Different formulations of the same pesticide can vary in toxicity.

4. Diagnosis hinges on a detailed exposure history and clinical signs. When the history is unclear, a high level of suspicion for pesticide poisoning is necessary.

5. Many pesticides have delayed onset of symptoms, making it crucial for patients with oral exposure to be monitored for a minimum of 6 to 48 hours, depending on the specific pesticide involved.

6. The management of acute pesticide poisoning prioritizes resuscitation and supportive care. Severe cases often require extended hospital stays, particularly in an intensive care unit (ICU).

7. The risk of secondary contamination in healthcare workers is minimal when universal precautions, such as the use of protective gloves, are observed.

8. The antidote for poisoning by anticholinesterase pesticides (organophosphates and carbamates) is atropine. It should be administered promptly and titrated based on the clinical response. Pralidoxime, while used in acute organophosphate poisoning, has limited supporting evidence and its efficacy remains inconclusive.

Introduction

Pesticide-related self-poisoning accounts for approximately 30% of suicides globally. While pesticides are generally more toxic than pharmaceuticals, not all exposures result in clinically significant poisoning. In countries like Australia, accidental pesticide exposure is common, though the majority of affected individuals do not require hospitalization.

Pesticide poisoning can result from both acute (such as intentional self-harm) and chronic (e.g., occupational) exposures. This chapter primarily addresses the acute exposure, which is of greater concern to emergency medical professionals.

A pesticide is defined as any substance used for controlling pests, including a wide variety of chemicals. These can be classified based on their intended target, such as insecticides, herbicides, fungicides, rodenticides, and nematicides. Other classification systems might focus on the chemical structure, toxicity to animals (LD50), or the mechanism of action.

Given the relatively low incidence of pesticide poisoning, healthcare professionals may not initially consider it in differential diagnoses. Case reports have demonstrated delayed diagnoses when pesticide poisoning was not suspected early on. This chapter specifically discusses agricultural chemicals in Australasia, especially insecticides like organophosphates (OPs) and carbamates. Table 25.15.3 provides a summary of the clinical signs and management strategies for various pesticides.

Aetiology and Pathophysiology

Acute pesticide poisoning typically requires hospitalization and ongoing care, especially in the case of intentional self-poisoning. However, significant poisoning can also occur due to accidental exposure, such as mishandling or improper storage of pesticides.

The pathophysiology of acute pesticide poisoning varies greatly depending on the specific compound involved. Many pesticides affect multiple systems in the body, but the exact mechanisms of toxicity are often poorly understood. Consequently, there is limited guidance for managing exposures.

Pesticide formulations can contain additional toxic agents, such as hydrocarbon-based solvents or surfactants, which enhance penetration into plants but may also increase human toxicity. In some cases, these co-formulants are more harmful than the active pesticide ingredient.

Epidemiology

Acute pesticide poisoning is a significant concern in developing nations, especially in the Asia-Pacific region. Organophosphate pesticides (OPs) are the leading cause of pesticide-related deaths globally. In developed countries, severe pesticide poisoning is rare but may still be more prevalent in rural areas where concentrated pesticide formulations are more accessible.

Prevention

Primary Exposure: Regulatory measures, such as limiting the availability of highly toxic pesticides, can help reduce the incidence of self-poisoning. In Australia, stringent regulations on chemicals like paraquat and organochlorines have resulted in a decrease in related fatalities. Proper pesticide storage, handling, and usage can prevent both intentional and accidental exposures.

Secondary Exposure (Nosocomial Poisoning)

Secondary exposure refers to the risk of healthcare workers or family members being poisoned by contact with a contaminated patient. Such cases are exceedingly rare but can occur if appropriate universal precautions are not followed. Mild symptoms may include nausea, dizziness, and headaches, which typically resolve with fresh air exposure. Proper decontamination procedures, including skin cleansing and disposal of contaminated clothing, are essential for preventing secondary poisoning.

Anticholinesterase Pesticides

Anticholinesterase pesticides, including organophosphates (OPs) and carbamates, are among the most commonly used pesticides. The clinical toxicity of these compounds is not fully understood, and even low-level exposures can result in significant poisoning. While carbamates are generally less toxic and their effects are shorter-lived than OPs, certain carbamates like carbofuran can still cause severe toxicity and even death.

Mechanism of Toxicity

The primary mechanism of toxicity for anticholinesterase compounds is the inhibition of acetylcholinesterase (AChE). AChE is an enzyme that normally breaks down acetylcholine at nerve synapses. When inhibited, acetylcholine accumulates, leading to overstimulation of cholinergic receptors, which disrupts normal nervous system function. This cascade of events causes a range of symptoms known as the "acute cholinergic crisis."

In organophosphate poisoning, the inhibition of AChE can sometimes be reversed if an oxime is administered soon after exposure. However, once the enzyme undergoes "ageing" (irreversible inhibition), AChE can no longer be reactivated. In contrast, carbamate exposure typically allows for spontaneous reactivation of AChE, and aging does not occur.

Clinical Features

The hallmark of anticholinesterase poisoning is the acute cholinergic crisis, characterized by a combination of symptoms affecting various organ systems, including gastrointestinal distress, respiratory failure, and neurological signs. The severity and duration of these symptoms depend on the specific pesticide involved and the extent of exposure.

Differential Diagnosis

When a history of exposure is not available, the differential diagnosis can include other causes of cholinergic symptoms, such as poisoning with clonidine, opioids, dopamine antagonists, or envenoming by funnel-web spiders. Pontine hemorrhage also presents with some similar clinical features.

Clinical Investigation

Diagnosis primarily relies on clinical presentation, though cholinesterase activity levels can be useful for confirmation. A decrease in cholinesterase activity within 6 hours of exposure suggests significant poisoning. In cases of severe poisoning, erythrocyte AChE activity drops below 20% of normal. Serial measurements of AChE can help monitor the effectiveness of treatment with oximes and confirm whether reactivation has occurred.

Criteria for Diagnosis

Acute anticholinesterase poisoning is diagnosed based on the patient's exposure history and clinical signs. A high index of suspicion is necessary, particularly when exposure details are unclear.

Acute pesticide poisoning can manifest in various ways depending on the type of pesticide involved, and the management of these cases requires timely and specific interventions. Here's a detailed analysis of common types of pesticide poisoning and their management:

Organophosphate (OP) and Carbamate Poisoning

Symptoms of OP and carbamate poisoning usually include acute cholinergic crisis, which is characterized by a range of muscarinic effects such as excessive salivation, sweating, and respiratory distress, as well as nicotinic effects like muscle weakness. Blood tests may show reduced acetylcholinesterase (AChE) activity, indicating significant exposure, and butyrylcholinesterase (BChE) levels can be used as a marker of exposure, though not necessarily toxicity severity. Initial management involves resuscitation and supportive care, including gastrointestinal decontamination and dermal cleansing. Atropine, a muscarinic antagonist, is used to reverse the muscarinic symptoms, and pralidoxime may be considered to reverse neuromuscular weakness, although its efficacy is debated.

Paraquat Poisoning

Paraquat poisoning typically presents with severe gastrointestinal symptoms and acute kidney injury (AKI), which may progress to pneumonitis, hepatotoxicity, and potentially death. Diagnosis can be confirmed through urinary dithionite testing. The management of paraquat poisoning requires supportive care, including intravenous rehydration to support renal excretion. Activated charcoal or Fuller's earth may be used if available, and early hemodialysis or hemoperfusion may be considered if the patient is seen within 2-4 hours of ingestion. Corticosteroids are sometimes used, though their efficacy is not always clear.

Glyphosate Poisoning

Glyphosate poisoning results in abdominal pain, nausea, vomiting, and diarrhea, which can progress to multiorgan dysfunction, including kidney failure and metabolic acidosis. Blood gas analysis, serum electrolytes, and kidney function tests are essential for monitoring. In mild cases, patients are managed with intravenous fluids and supportive care. For more severe cases, including those with acute kidney injury, the use of hemodialysis may be necessary.

MCPA, 2,4-D, and Bromoxynil Poisoning

Symptoms of poisoning with these herbicides include gastrointestinal distress, myalgia, rhabdomyolysis, hyperthermia, and neurological symptoms such as agitation and confusion. Blood gases typically show respiratory alkalosis followed by metabolic acidosis. Management focuses on supportive care, including monitoring vital signs and electrolyte balance, as well as gastrointestinal decontamination with activated charcoal. If the patient's acid-base balance deteriorates, urinary alkalinization and, in severe cases, hemodialysis, may be required.

Herbicide Poisoning (Propanil, Metolachlor, Glufosinate)

Poisoning with amide herbicides such as propanil and metolachlor causes gastrointestinal distress, agitation, seizures, and acidosis, and may lead to methemoglobinemia and haemolysis in the case of propanil. In severe cases, propanil poisoning may require methylene blue for treatment of methemoglobinemia. Glufosinate poisoning, on the other hand, can lead to seizures, coma, and respiratory failure. Treatment includes supportive care, with an emphasis on fluid management to ensure adequate urine output, and early referral for hemodialysis in cases of kidney impairment.

General Treatment and Management

In all cases of acute pesticide poisoning, initial treatment focuses on stabilizing the patient by managing the airway, breathing, and circulation. Resuscitation is crucial, especially in cases of severe poisoning. For patients with significant exposure, decontamination is an essential first step, which may involve removing contaminated clothing, performing dermal decontamination with soap and water, and gastrointestinal decontamination with activated charcoal if the patient presents early after ingestion. Continuous monitoring is necessary, and for those with severe poisoning, intensive care may be required.

Antidotes and Further Interventions

Atropine is commonly used to counteract the muscarinic effects of organophosphates and carbamates. Oximes, such as pralidoxime, are used to treat neuromuscular symptoms by reactivating acetylcholinesterase, although their use and effectiveness remain controversial. In cases of severe poisoning, benzodiazepines may be used to manage seizures, and specific antidotes for methemoglobinemia (such as methylene blue) or other complications may also be necessary.

Prognosis

The prognosis for patients with pesticide poisoning varies depending on the type of pesticide, the severity of exposure, and the timeliness of treatment. Mortality rates are generally higher for organophosphate poisoning, especially in severe cases, and can exceed 10%. However, the prognosis improves significantly for dermal exposures, which typically result in less severe toxicity.

In conclusion, the treatment of acute pesticide poisoning is highly dependent on the specific pesticide involved and the severity of the poisoning. Early intervention, including decontamination, resuscitation, and the use of appropriate antidotes, is key to improving patient outcomes. However, further research is necessary to refine treatment protocols and optimize the use of antidotes like oximes.

Chapter 16
Herbicides

This chapter highlights the diverse toxicity profiles of common herbicides and the challenges in managing acute poisoning cases.

1. Paraquat Poisoning

Acute paraquat ingestion has a high fatality rate due to rapid multi-organ failure or delayed pulmonary fibrosis.

Ingestion of even a small amount (e.g., a single mouthful of 20% w/v solution) is often lethal.

Currently, no effective treatment options are available for paraquat poisoning.

2. Glyphosate-Containing Herbicides

The surfactant co-formulant or its salt is believed to be the primary toxic component in glyphosate-based herbicides.

Although the exact mechanism of toxicity remains unclear, severe cases are linked to multi-organ damage and metabolic acidosis.

Management involves supportive care to address systemic effects.

3. Chlorophenoxy Herbicides

Herbicides like 2-methyl-4-chlorophenoxyacetic acid generally result in mild toxicity.

However, fatalities can occur due to the uncoupling of oxidative phosphorylation.

Toxicity significantly increases when herbicides are combined with bromoxynil in co-formulations.

Introduction

Herbicide poisoning can lead to significant morbidity and mortality, particularly in cases involving toxic substances like paraquat. These herbicides, though not common in developed countries, are a considerable cause of mortality in developing nations. The severity of poisoning varies depending on the herbicide type, with some causing severe multi-organ damage and others presenting less dangerous toxicity.

Paraquat Poisoning

Paraquat is a potent, non-selective herbicide that is highly toxic when ingested, with mortality rates ranging from 50% to 90%. This is primarily due to rapid multi-organ failure or delayed progressive pulmonary fibrosis. Ingestion of as little as 20 mL of a 20% solution can be fatal. Although access to paraquat is tightly controlled in countries like Australia, it remains a significant cause of death in parts of

Asia. Notably, paraquat is minimally absorbed through inhalation or intact skin, limiting exposure through these routes.

Toxic Mechanism

Paraquat toxicity arises from the production of free oxygen radicals, which cause oxidative damage to cells. The herbicide accumulates in high concentrations in the lungs and kidneys due to active uptake in the type II pneumocytes and renal tubular cells. The free radicals generated lead to lipid peroxidation, mitochondrial dysfunction, and cell death, resulting in widespread tissue damage. This mechanism leads to the characteristic multi-organ failure seen in severe poisoning cases.

Clinical Features

After ingestion, patients typically experience gastrointestinal distress, including nausea, vomiting, and diarrhea. Within hours, oral mucosal ulceration and potential esophageal perforation can occur. Those who ingest more than 20 mL often develop severe systemic toxicity, including pneumonitis, liver and kidney dysfunction, hypotension, and acute kidney injury. Respiratory failure, due to pulmonary fibrosis, is the primary cause of death, although death can also be delayed in patients who ingest smaller amounts (less than 20 mL), with death potentially occurring weeks or months after ingestion due to complications. In contrast, Diquat, another bipyridyl herbicide, does not accumulate in the lungs as significantly and is less likely to cause delayed pulmonary fibrosis.

Clinical Investigations

To confirm paraquat exposure, a urinary dithionite test is performed. The test involves adding a sodium dithionite solution to urine, where a blue color indicates paraquat ingestion, and a green color indicates diquat. The intensity of the color change correlates with the concentration of paraquat. A negative result after six hours suggests that significant exposure is unlikely. Further tests should focus on monitoring organ function, particularly the kidneys, liver, and lungs. Serial blood gas measurements and chest X-rays can assess pulmonary injury, while CT scans can help in diagnosing pulmonary fibrosis.

Differential Diagnosis

Acute paraquat poisoning may resemble other toxic exposures, such as sepsis or poisoning with substances like phosphine, colchicine, or iron. However, the presence of marked oropharyngeal necrosis is a distinguishing feature of paraquat poisoning.

Treatment

Treatment for paraquat poisoning primarily focuses on supportive care. All patients with suspected paraquat ingestion should be monitored in a hospital for at least 12 hours due to the potential for severe toxicity. Initial treatment includes hydration to support renal function and facilitate the elimination of paraquat from the body.

For severe poisoning, especially within the first 24 hours, treatment becomes largely palliative, as these patients have a very low chance of survival. For patients presenting with significant systemic toxicity (e.g., hypotension, hypoxia, acidosis, or low Glasgow Coma Scale score), early palliative care is recommended.

Decontamination

For patients who present within 2 hours of ingestion, decontamination using activated charcoal or Fuller's earth can help reduce further absorption of the toxin.

Immunosuppression

Some treatment regimens attempt to mitigate the inflammatory response triggered by paraquat poisoning. Immunosuppressive therapies, such as cyclophosphamide and corticosteroids (e.g., methylprednisolone and dexamethasone), have shown promise in small clinical trials. A recent randomized controlled trial (RCT) investigating high-dose immunosuppression suggested some benefit in improving survival rates, but the evidence remains inconclusive.

Enhanced Elimination

In cases of severe poisoning, procedures to enhance elimination, such as hemodialysis, may be considered to help clear the paraquat from the bloodstream more quickly. However, the utility of this approach remains a subject of ongoing research.

Urinary Dithionite Test for Paraquat Poisoning

The urinary dithionite test is a valuable diagnostic tool used to confirm significant paraquat exposure, which can guide further management decisions. This test, available for free distribution by Syngenta in Australia and several other countries, involves analyzing a urine sample for a color change. A blue color indicates paraquat ingestion, while a green color suggests diquat ingestion. The intensity of the color change is directly correlated with the concentration of the ingested substance, with darker shades indicating higher concentrations. If the test returns negative results within six hours post-ingestion, it suggests that the exposure is likely not significant.

Immunosuppressive Therapy and Supportive Care in Paraquat Poisoning

A study comparing the effects of immunosuppressive therapy (cyclophosphamide and intravenous methylprednisolone followed by oral dexamethasone) to standard care, including fluids, charcoal, and analgesia, found that immunosuppressive therapy did not significantly improve survival rates. However, the study noted a potentially beneficial effect of a two-week course of dexamethasone, though this requires further research. A recommended regimen for immunosuppressive treatment includes methylprednisolone 1g/day for three days, followed by a five-week course of dexamethasone at 8 mg three times daily.

Antioxidant Treatment for Paraquat Poisoning

Several antioxidants, including acetylcysteine, salicylic acid, vitamin C, and vitamin E, have been suggested as potential treatments for paraquat poisoning. These antioxidants theoretically counteract oxidative stress caused by paraquat's free radical production. While the optimal dosing regimens are not yet established, for acetylcysteine, the same dosing used for paracetamol overdose is employed: a loading dose of 200 mg/kg over four hours, followed by 150 mg/kg/day for seven days.

Enhanced Elimination Techniques for Paraquat

The use of hemodialysis or hemoperfusion to enhance the elimination of paraquat is debated. Paraquat is rapidly excreted unchanged in the urine within 12 to 24 hours, making additional elimination methods potentially of limited value. Animal studies suggest that hemoperfusion is most effective when initiated within two hours of ingestion. Some studies indicate that early hemodialysis or hemoperfusion may reduce mortality, but these studies have methodological limitations. If available, early hemodialysis should be considered, with intermittent hemodialysis being the preferred modality.

Prognosis of Paraquat Poisoning

The prognosis of paraquat poisoning is primarily determined by the amount ingested. Ingestions exceeding 50 to 100 mL of concentrated paraquat (>20% w/v) typically result in rapid, severe organ failure. Smaller ingestions cause acute kidney and lung injury within the first week, often leading to progressive pulmonary fibrosis. The mortality rate from pulmonary fibrosis can exceed 50%, with symptoms sometimes appearing up to six weeks after ingestion. Poor prognostic indicators include the development of renal failure, chest x-ray abnormalities, and a burning sensation on the skin. Plasma paraquat levels, when available, may be used to predict prognosis, but such assays are not accessible in all regions.

Glyphosate Poisoning

Glyphosate, a widely used herbicide, is available in two common formulations: ready-to-use (1% to 5%) and concentrated (30% to 50%). Glyphosate is absorbed through the gastrointestinal tract, and ingestion is the primary route of poisoning. Symptoms can vary from mild gastrointestinal discomfort after ingestion of dilute solutions to severe poisoning from concentrated solutions, which may lead to life-threatening conditions such as corrosive gastrointestinal injury, metabolic acidosis, renal failure, and pneumonitis. Severe poisoning can progress to multi-organ failure, shock, and death within 12 to 72 hours.

Mechanism of Glyphosate Toxicity

Glyphosate itself exhibits minimal toxicity to mammals. However, the surfactants used in glyphosate formulations, such as polyoxyethyleneamine (POEA), contribute significantly to its toxicity. POEA can disrupt cellular membranes and uncouple oxidative phosphorylation. In some formulations, severe hyperkalemia can also occur, particularly with potassium-based glyphosate salts.

Clinical Features of Glyphosate Poisoning

The clinical presentation of glyphosate poisoning varies. After ingestion of diluted solutions, mild gastrointestinal symptoms may resolve without medical intervention. However, ingestion of concentrated glyphosate can result in severe toxicity characterized by gastrointestinal injury, electrolyte imbalances, metabolic acidosis, hypotension, renal failure, and pneumonitis. This may progress to multi-organ failure, shock, and death.

Diagnosis and Investigation in Glyphosate Poisoning

Diagnosis primarily relies on a history of exposure, making it crucial to maintain a high index of suspicion. There are no specific diagnostic tests for glyphosate poisoning, although serial blood gases and biochemistry can help identify acidosis, hyperkalemia, and renal impairment. A chest x-ray is recommended if there is concern for pneumonitis or pulmonary edema. Glyphosate concentration assays, which may correlate with outcomes, are not widely available.

Treatment of Glyphosate Poisoning

The management of glyphosate poisoning is largely supportive. Intravenous fluids should be used to replace gastrointestinal losses, and biochemical and acid-base abnormalities should be corrected. In cases of severe poisoning, dialysis may be considered for acidosis, hyperkalemia, or renal failure. All patients should be observed for at least six hours after ingestion, with a longer observation period recommended for those with gastrointestinal symptoms, which may worsen over time.

Prognosis of Glyphosate Poisoning

The prognosis of glyphosate poisoning depends on the severity of exposure and the presence of complications. Elderly patients and those with metabolic acidosis, hyperkalemia, or end-organ dysfunction have a worse prognosis. Mortality rates vary, but a Sri Lankan study found a mortality rate of 3.2% in cases of acute poisoning with glyphosate-containing herbicides.

Chlorophenoxy Herbicides Poisoning

herbicides, such as MCPA, 2,4-D, and mecoprop, are selective herbicides that primarily affect broad-leaved plants. These herbicides are often combined with other chemicals, which can increase toxicity. herbicides primarily cause gastrointestinal irritation, with more severe toxicity being less common. A study of 181 patients in Sri Lanka found that 85% of those who ingested MCPA experienced minimal symptoms. However, co-formulations containing bromoxynil can be significantly more toxic due to the potential for mitochondrial uncoupling, leading to metabolic acidosis, hyperthermia, and multi-organ failure.

Treatment of Chlorophenoxy Herbicides Poisoning

Activated charcoal should be administered early for decontamination. Patients should be monitored for at least six hours after ingestion, with extended observation for those who ingest bromoxynil-containing formulations due to the delayed onset of toxicity. Standard supportive care includes maintaining hydration, and urinary alkalinization may be helpful in more severe cases of MCPA poisoning. Early dialysis may be necessary to manage metabolic acidosis in cases of bromoxynil poisoning, although it does not significantly clear the toxins.

Controversies in Herbicide Poisoning Management

Paraquat: The debate continues regarding whether early palliation or aggressive treatment is more beneficial for patients with large paraquat ingestions. The effectiveness and dosing of anti-inflammatory drugs and antioxidants are also under investigation.

Glyphosate: There is ongoing discussion about the relative contributions of glyphosate, its salts, and other co-formulants to the severity of poisoning. Additionally, the clinical and analytical predictors for severe poisoning are still being studied.

Chlorophenoxy Herbicides: The role of co-formulants such as bromoxynil in enhancing toxicity remains controversial, with some studies suggesting they significantly increase the risk of severe outcomes.

Chapter 17
Ethanol and Other Toxic Alcohols

Key Considerations

1. Impact on Health: Ethanol significantly contributes to morbidity, mortality, and frequent emergency department (ED) visits in Western societies, often stemming from acute intoxication, withdrawal, or complications of chronic use.

2. CNS Effects: Ethanol's central nervous system (CNS) depressant effects can amplify those of other depressants and become life-threatening without intervention.

3. Withdrawal Risks: Ethanol withdrawal is a critical condition with a mortality rate of up to 5% in the absence of medical treatment.

4. Wernicke Encephalopathy (WE): Often underdiagnosed, WE requires prompt

recognition and treatment with intravenous thiamine, especially in patients with prolonged alcohol abuse and altered mental status.

5. Toxic Alcohols: Methanol and ethylene glycol, even in small amounts, are lethal due to toxic metabolite production. Dialysis is the preferred treatment.

6. Diagnostic Challenges: Elevated anion-gap metabolic acidosis with a raised osmolar gap signals severe toxicity in toxic alcohol ingestion. However, the osmolar gap alone lacks sensitivity and cannot exclude toxic alcohol poisoning.

Introduction

Alcohols are hydrocarbons containing a hydroxyl group (-OH). Among them, ethanol is the most prevalent recreational substance in Australasia and Western societies, where misuse leads to substantial mortality and morbidity. For instance, an estimated 3,290 alcohol-related deaths and over 72,000 hospitalizations occurred in Australia in 1997. Approximately 10% of ED presentations in Australia are alcohol-related.

This chapter focuses on acute ethanol intoxication, withdrawal, and specific emergencies like Wernicke encephalopathy (WE) and alcoholic ketoacidosis (AKA). Toxic alcohols such as methanol and ethylene glycol, though less frequently encountered, pose life-threatening risks when ingested and require early intervention.

Ethanol

Pharmacology

Ethanol, a small molecule absorbed from the stomach and intestines, is distributed in total body water due to its water and lipid solubility. While most ethanol undergoes hepatic metabolism, a small fraction is excreted unchanged through the lungs, kidneys, and sweat.

Metabolism: Ethanol is oxidized by alcohol dehydrogenases (ADH) into acetaldehyde, then metabolized to acetate by aldehyde dehydrogenase. Acetate enters the Krebs cycle for conversion to water and carbon dioxide. Adequate thiamine levels are crucial for these processes.

Kinetics: At low ethanol concentrations, metabolism follows first-order kinetics, but shifts to zero-order kinetics at higher levels due to saturation of ADH enzymes. Chronic alcohol use enhances metabolism via the microsomal ethanol oxidizing system.

Clinical Presentation

Acute Intoxication:
Symptoms of acute intoxication are dose-dependent but vary based on individual tolerance. They progress from initial euphoria and disinhibition to impaired judgment, motor

dysfunction, emotional instability, and, at higher levels, coma, respiratory depression, or death.

ED Presentations: Alcohol intoxication frequently accompanies trauma, violence, self-harm, and social emergencies. It is often misattributed as the sole cause of altered mental states, masking coexisting conditions. Diagnosis is confirmed via breath or blood ethanol levels.

Ethanol Withdrawal Syndrome:
Withdrawal symptoms occur within 6–24 hours of reduced intake in dependent individuals, peaking at 50 hours. Without treatment, mortality can reach 5%.

Mild Symptoms: Nausea, tremors, tachycardia, and anxiety due to mild autonomic hyperactivity.

Severe Symptoms: Hallucinations, seizures, delirium tremens, and autonomic instability in advanced cases.

Wernicke Encephalopathy (WE)

A neurological emergency caused by thiamine deficiency in chronic alcohol users, WE is underdiagnosed and carries a 10–20% mortality rate without treatment.

Classic Triad: Oculomotor disturbances (e.g., nystagmus), altered mental status, and ataxia, though less than 20% of cases present with all three.

Management: Administer parenteral thiamine immediately upon suspicion to prevent progression to irreversible neurological damage.

Alcoholic Ketoacidosis (AKA)

AKA is a metabolic complication triggered by prolonged heavy drinking followed by a period of fasting, leading to a ketoacidotic state.

Pathophysiology: Starvation-induced gluconeogenesis shifts to lactate production in alcoholics, increasing fatty acid metabolism and ketoacid accumulation.

Presentation: Patients report nausea, vomiting, abdominal pain, and may have been misdiagnosed with "alcoholic gastritis" or "query pancreatitis" in prior episodes.

Differential Diagnosis: Unlike diabetic ketoacidosis, AKA typically presents with normal mental status and lacks the pronounced alterations in consciousness seen in toxic alcohol poisoning.

Toxic Alcohol Poisoning

Methanol and ethylene glycol ingestion lead to the production of toxic metabolites causing acidosis and organ failure.

Clinical Indicators: Elevated anion-gap metabolic acidosis and osmolar gap are diagnostic hallmarks. Methanol affects vision, while ethylene glycol causes renal damage and crystalluria.

Management: Dialysis is the definitive treatment to remove toxic metabolites and correct acid-base imbalances.

Investigations

Ethanol Levels: Breath and blood ethanol measurements confirm intoxication but cannot exclude coexisting pathology.

Laboratory Findings in AKA: Low or absent ethanol levels, normal/low glucose, high anion-gap acidosis, and undetectable or low urinary ketones.

Treatment

Acute Ethanol Intoxication

Supportive care is critical, focusing on airway protection, fluid resuscitation, and maintaining normoglycemia. Administer intravenous thiamine to prevent complications like WE.

Ethanol Withdrawal

Prompt recognition and medical intervention, including benzodiazepines for symptom control, are essential to manage withdrawal and prevent complications like delirium tremens.

Toxic Alcohol Poisoning

Immediate treatment involves fomepizole or ethanol to inhibit alcohol dehydrogenase, followed by hemodialysis to remove toxic metabolites.

Summary: Thiamine Administration Guidelines in Clinical Practice

Administration and Dosage

Standard Administration: Thiamine is diluted in 100 mL of 0.9% saline and infused over 60 minutes.

Discretionary Use: In the absence of clear evidence of chronic alcohol misuse, thiamine administration is guided by clinician discretion.

Acute Alcohol Intoxication: In cases of suspected chronic alcohol abuse, 200 mg IV stat is the recommended dose.

Indications and Clinical Scenarios

1. Suspected Wernicke's Encephalopathy (WE)

Criteria: Presence of one or more of the following:

Acute confusion or memory disturbance

Ataxia, nystagmus, ophthalmoplegia

Unexplained hypotension or hypothermia

Reduced consciousness or coma

Treatment Protocol:

Administer 500 mg thiamine IV three times daily (tds) if WE is strongly suspected, per senior clinician discretion.

Continue for up to three days, reassessing daily.

2. Altered Mental Status (Any Cause) with Suspected Chronic Alcohol Abuse:

Protocol: Administer 200 mg IV tds until mental status normalizes, with dose review after three days.

3. Acute Alcohol Withdrawal Without Mental Status Changes:

Signs of Withdrawal:

Anxiety, agitation, insomnia

Tremors, tachycardia, hypertension

Sweating, sensory distortions, fever without infection

Protocol:

Administer 200 mg IV tds for 24 hours, then reassess dosage.

Supportive Management

Serum Magnesium: Check and replace if levels are subnormal.

Glucose Supplementation: Administer post-thiamine infusion to prevent worsening neurological injury.

Alcohol Withdrawal Scale (AWS): Use for monitoring and diazepam administration per protocol for withdrawal management.

Referral Considerations: Involve drug and alcohol services when clinically appropriate to support rehabilitation.

Thiamine Therapy Outcomes in Wernicke's Encephalopathy

Early Intervention: Neurological symptoms like ophthalmoplegia and nystagmus typically respond within hours to days.

Prognostic Challenges: Ataxia and cognitive changes show slower recovery, with up to 50% of cases experiencing incomplete resolution despite treatment.

Supplementation Needs: Concurrent magnesium replacement is critical for optimal recovery.

Clinical Implications of Ethanol-Related Presentations

Patients presenting with ethanol-related complications, such as ketoacidosis or withdrawal syndromes, require comprehensive management:

Ketoacidosis: Address with thiamine, dextrose, and electrolyte monitoring to prevent progression.

Severe Withdrawal: Admit to a safe environment, such as an intensive care unit, for those requiring airway or cardiovascular support.

Expert Recommendations for Toxic Alcohol Exposure

Diagnosis Challenges: Methanol and ethylene glycol ingestion should be suspected in patients with unexplained high anion-gap metabolic acidosis or osmolar gap.

Laboratory Analysis: Direct assays, when available, expedite diagnosis but are rarely accessible.

Treatment Protocols:

Administer ethanol or fomepizole to inhibit toxic metabolite formation.

Provide intensive monitoring for acid-base disturbances and organ dysfunction.

Chapter 18
Carbon Monoxide Poisoning

Key Considerations

1. Prevalence: Carbon monoxide (CO) poisoning is the leading cause of fatal poisoning-related suicides in Australia and the United Kingdom.

2. Sources: It is generated by incomplete combustion and is present in car exhaust, malfunctioning heaters, fires, and some industrial environments.

3. Neuropsychological Impact: CO poisoning can result in long-lasting neuropsychological damage.

4. Oxygen Therapy: High concentrations of oxygen accelerate the elimination of CO, with efficacy increasing in proportion to inspired oxygen pressure.

5. Therapeutic Approaches: The optimal method of oxygen administration for improved clinical outcomes remains debated.

Introduction

Carbon monoxide poisoning is a significant cause of morbidity and mortality globally. Prompt intervention with 100% oxygen therapy is the cornerstone of management and often results in favorable outcomes. However, the efficacy of additional therapies in mitigating the risk of long-term neurological damage remains uncertain.

Aetiology, Pathophysiology, and Pathology

Characteristics and Sources: CO is a colorless, odorless, tasteless, and non-irritating gas produced by incomplete hydrocarbon combustion. While trace amounts are endogenously produced in metabolic processes, significant exposure arises from sources like vehicle exhaust, fires, cigarette smoke, and faulty heating appliances. Advanced catalytic converters in modern vehicles have markedly reduced CO emissions.

Pathophysiology

CO binds to hemoglobin with an affinity 210 times greater than oxygen, impairing oxygen transport. Beyond this, CO disrupts cellular oxidative functions, interacts with myoglobin and cytochrome oxidase, and causes lipid peroxidation in the brain. This cascade results in tissue hypoxia, culminating in varying levels of organ damage or death depending on exposure duration, ambient CO levels, and individual health status.

Epidemiology

Globally, CO poisoning is a critical public health issue, contributing to both accidental and intentional injuries. In the United States, CO poisoning accounts for 1,000–2,000 deaths annually from approximately 40,000 exposures. In regions like East Asia, charcoal-burning suicides have become increasingly prevalent.

Prevention

Preventative measures include CO monitors in environments prone to high exposure and the widespread use of catalytic converters in vehicles. These advancements have significantly reduced fatal CO poisoning rates in some regions.

Clinical Features

Symptoms and Signs: The clinical presentation of CO poisoning varies with carboxyhemoglobin (COHb) levels. Early symptoms are nonspecific, such as headache, dizziness, and nausea, while severe poisoning manifests as confusion, arrhythmias, and loss of consciousness. Death ensues when cardiac hypoxia prevents compensatory mechanisms.

Special Populations

Pregnant Women: Fetal hemoglobin's high CO affinity makes fetuses especially vulnerable, often resulting in death or neurological impairment.

Long-Term Effects: Persistent neuropsychiatric sequelae, such as memory deficits and mood disorders, are common, particularly in patients who experienced prolonged unconsciousness during poisoning.

Diagnosis

Differential Diagnosis: In suspected suicides, additional toxic substances should be considered. Smoke inhalation victims often concurrently suffer cyanide poisoning, which may exacerbate symptoms disproportionate to COHb levels.

Clinical Investigations

Blood Gases and Oximetry: COHb levels confirm acute CO exposure but are unreliable predictors of severity or prognosis due to individual variations and oxygen administration prior to testing.

ECG: A baseline and follow-up ECG (at 6 and 24 hours) are essential to detect cardiac ischemia or arrhythmias. Elevated troponin levels correlate with increased long-term mortality.

Treatment

Immediate Management: Stabilizing the airway, providing 100% oxygen, and monitoring cardiac and neurological function are critical. Patients with impaired consciousness may require intubation and mechanical ventilation.

Oxygen Therapy: Administering 100% oxygen reduces COHb's half-life from four hours in ambient air to 40 minutes. Hyperbaric oxygen therapy (HBO), when accessible, accelerates this further to 20 minutes and improves tissue oxygenation. The use of HBO is most appropriate for patients at high risk of long-term neurological sequelae.

Supportive Measures: Correcting metabolic acidosis and electrolyte imbalances, monitoring for myocardial damage, and ensuring adequate rest are integral components of care.

Prognosis

The majority of patients recover well with timely oxygen therapy. However, delayed neuropsychiatric effects, including memory impairment and mood disturbances, necessitate long-term follow-up and rehabilitation in severe cases.

Controversies

1. Debate on Benefits and Risks of Hyperbaric Oxygen Therapy (HBO):
A primary point of contention surrounds the benefits, risks, and clinical indications for hyperbaric oxygen therapy (HBO). Efforts to address this uncertainty through further clinical trials may face challenges due to strong convictions held by certain HBO practitioners. Eight randomized clinical trials (RCTs) have produced highly conflicting results. Some studies suggest HBO may have harmful effects, while others argue it offers significant benefits. Systematic reviews, however, have failed to demonstrate a clear advantage of HBO, citing evidence of various biases in trials reporting positive outcomes. Conversely, negative trials often suffered from methodological issues such as low follow-up rates, unconventional control interventions, and the inclusion of patients with less severe poisoning.

2. Use of HBO in Clinical Practice:
In facilities equipped with hyperbaric chambers, HBO may be considered justifiable if it can be administered promptly and safely. Its biological rationale lies in its ability to rapidly increase oxygen delivery and eliminate carbon monoxide. However, transferring patients between hospitals for delayed HBO treatment—particularly over long distances—lacks support from current RCT evidence, animal studies, and the established pathophysiology of carbon monoxide poisoning.

3. Role of Biomarkers in Prognosis:
There is growing interest in utilizing the measurement of the S100B protein as a prognostic tool in patients undergoing evaluation for carbon monoxide poisoning.

Chapter 19
Anticonvulsants

Key Considerations

1. CNS Effects in Overdose: Anticonvulsant overdoses predominantly affect the central nervous system (CNS), but certain agents can also cause significant cardiotoxicity.

2. Activated Charcoal: Administering multiple doses of activated charcoal can effectively reduce the duration of toxicity in carbamazepine and phenytoin overdoses.

3. Serum Concentrations: Serum drug levels often correlate with clinical toxicity, particularly for carbamazepine and phenytoin, guiding treatment in severe cases.

4. Extracorporeal Elimination: Severe toxicity may necessitate extracorporeal elimination, depending on the specific agent involved.

5. Paradoxical Seizures: Although uncommon, paradoxical seizures can occur with any anticonvulsant, including phenytoin.

Introduction

While anticonvulsants are primarily used to treat seizure disorders, their indications now include managing pain and mood disorders. This broader use has led to increased cases of poisoning from these medications. This chapter examines common toxicities related to anticonvulsants, focusing on carbamazepine, phenytoin, and sodium valproate.

Carbamazepine

Pathophysiology

Carbamazepine, structurally related to tricyclic antidepressants, blocks voltage-gated sodium channels in the CNS and inhibits N-methyl-D-aspartate (NMDA) and adenosine receptors. Its slow and incomplete absorption, along with its property of inducing its own metabolism, complicates its pharmacokinetics. Chronic use leads to faster drug clearance, reducing toxicity symptoms compared to drug-naive individuals. In overdose, prolonged half-lives are common due to delayed absorption and impaired elimination.

Clinical Features

Symptoms are primarily neurological, cardiovascular, and anticholinergic:

Neurological: Altered mental status, dysarthria, ataxia, seizures, and in severe cases, coma with respiratory depression.

Cardiovascular: Sinus tachycardia, hypotension, myocardial depression, atrioventricular block, and QRS prolongation.

Anticholinergic: Impaired gut motility leading to prolonged absorption, especially in sustained-release formulations.

Investigations

Key assessments include:

Blood sugar levels.

Serum carbamazepine concentrations to confirm toxicity and guide therapy.

ECG to monitor cardiac conduction abnormalities.

Toxicity is associated with:

Neurological symptoms at levels >10 mg/L (50 μmol/L).

Severe cardiac effects at levels >45 mg/L (200 μmol/L).

Treatment

Management involves:

1. Supportive Care: Prioritizing airway management and adequate monitoring.

2. Activated Charcoal: Early administration (50 g) can limit absorption, especially in significant ingestions (>20 mg/kg).

3. Multiple-Dose Activated Charcoal (MDAC): Recommended for persistent coma, typically administered every 4 hours until clinical improvement.

4. Sodium Bicarbonate: Administered for ventricular dysrhythmias caused by sodium channel blockade.

5. Extracorporeal Elimination: Indicated for severe cases with persistent coma, refractory seizures, or life-threatening dysrhythmias.

Patients ingesting >50 mg/kg require close monitoring in a resuscitation bay, while asymptomatic adults after 8 hours of observation may not need further intervention.

Phenytoin

Pathophysiology

Phenytoin inhibits voltage-dependent sodium channels, reducing neuronal excitability. In overdose, its absorption and metabolism become erratic and prolonged. Chronic toxicity often arises from dosing errors or drug interactions. Genetic polymorphisms in cytochrome P450 2C9 may delay drug clearance in some individuals, leading to severe toxicity.

Clinical Features

Neurological Symptoms: Ataxia, dysarthria, nystagmus, and, rarely, seizures or coma in massive overdoses (>100 mg/kg).

Other Effects: Hypernatremia, hyperglycemia, and hyperosmotic non-ketotic coma.

Cardiovascular Symptoms: Associated with rapid intravenous administration due to propylene glycol diluent rather than the drug itself.

Investigations

Serum phenytoin concentrations guide management:

Mild to moderate toxicity occurs at 20-50 mg/L.

Severe toxicity (coma, ataxia) correlates with levels >50 mg/L (200 μmol/L).

Treatment

Key interventions include:

1. Supportive Care: Maintaining airway safety and appropriate monitoring.

2. Activated Charcoal: Useful within 4 hours of significant overdose.

3. MDAC: Administered every 2-4 hours for unresolved toxicity, particularly in patients with genetic metabolic polymorphisms.

4. Extracorporeal Elimination: Employed for refractory cases with prolonged toxicity or seizures.

Patients with mild toxicity may be observed on a ward, while severe cases require intensive care.

Sodium Valproate

Pathophysiology

Sodium valproate increases gamma-aminobutyric acid (GABA) levels, modulating CNS excitability. In overdose, it disrupts mitochondrial metabolism and exhibits saturable protein binding, making it dialyzable. Toxicity severity correlates with the ingested dose:

<200 mg/kg: Mild sedation.

200-400 mg/kg: Profound CNS depression.

> 1000 mg/kg: Lethal effects such as multi-organ failure and cerebral edema.

Clinical Features

Toxicity manifests in various systems:

CNS: Coma, ataxia, seizures, cerebral edema.

Gastrointestinal: Nausea, vomiting, abdominal pain.

Cardiovascular and Hematological Effects: Rare but possible.

Investigations

Assess serum valproate levels to predict toxicity severity and guide treatment.

Treatment

1. Supportive Care: Monitoring airway, breathing, and circulation.

2. Activated Charcoal: Early use for significant ingestions.

3. Extracorporeal Elimination: Effective in severe toxicity due to its dialyzable nature.

Conclusion

Anticonvulsant overdoses necessitate a structured approach to diagnosis and management, focusing on the specific pharmacological properties of the agent involved. Timely investigations, supportive care, and targeted therapies such as activated charcoal and extracorporeal elimination can mitigate complications and improve outcomes.

References

1. Weaver LK. Carbon monoxide poisoning. Critical Care Clinics. 1999;15:297–317.

2. Chiew A, Buckley NA. Advances in carbon monoxide poisoning management. Critical Care. 2014;18(2):221.

3. Hampson NB. Trends in emergency department visits for carbon monoxide poisoning in the Pacific Northwest. Journal of Emergency Medicine. 1998;16:695–698.

4. Amos T, Appleby L, Kiernan K. Shifts in suicide methods: Car exhaust asphyxiation in England and Wales. Psychological Medicine. 2001;31:935–939.

5. Mott JA, Wolfe MI, Alverson CJ. Impact of national vehicle emission policies on declining US carbon monoxide-related mortality. JAMA. 2002;288:988–995.

6. Buckley NA, Dawson AH, Whyte IM. Hypertox: Assessment and treatment of poisoning. Hypertox Resource; 2012. Accessed August 2012.

7. Lippi G, Rastelli G, Meschi T. Cardiac implications of carbon monoxide poisoning: Clinical insights. Clinical Biochemistry. 2012;45:1278–1285.

8. Ahn KT, Park JH, Kim MS. Left ventricular systolic dysfunction prevalence and outcomes after carbon monoxide poisoning. International Journal of Cardiology. 2011;153:108–110.

9. Henry CR, Satran D, Lindgren B. Myocardial injury and its long-term impact post carbon monoxide poisoning. JAMA. 2006;295:398–402.

10. Pepe G, Castelli M, Nazerian P. Risk factors for delayed neuropsychological sequelae following carbon monoxide poisoning: A retrospective analysis. Scandinavian Journal of Trauma, Resuscitation and Emergency Medicine. 2011;19:16.

11. Ghannoum M, Yates C, Galvao TF, et al. Extracorporeal treatment for carbamazepine

poisoning: Systematic recommendations from EXTRIP. Clinical Toxicology (Philadelphia). 2014;52(10):993–1004.

12. Chan BS, Sellors K, Chiew AL, et al. Multidose activated charcoal in phenytoin toxicity linked to genetic polymorphism. Clinical Toxicology (Philadelphia). 2015;53(2):131–133.

13. Anseeuw K, Mowry JB, Burdmann EA, et al. Extracorporeal treatment in phenytoin toxicity: EXTRIP guidelines. American Journal of Kidney Diseases. 2016;67(2):187–197.

14. Ghannoum M, Laliberté M, Nolin TD, et al. Valproic acid poisoning and extracorporeal treatment: EXTRIP recommendations. Clinical Toxicology (Philadelphia). 2015;53(5):454–465.

15. Willis B, Reynolds P, Chu E, et al. Outcomes in overdoses of newer anticonvulsants: A poison center observational study. Journal of Medical

Toxicology. 2014;10:254–260. https://doi.org/10.1007/s13181-014-0384-5.

16. Alyahya B, Friesen M, Nauche B, Laliberté M. Acute lamotrigine overdose: A systematic review of adult and pediatric cases. Clinical Toxicology (Philadelphia). 2018;56(2):81–89. https://doi.org/10.1080/15563650.2017.1370096.

17. Lee T, Warrick BJ, Sarangarm P, et al. Levetiracetam in toxic seizures: Clinical evaluation. Clinical Toxicology (Philadelphia). 2018;56(3):175–181.
https://doi.org/10.1080/15563650.2017.1355056.

18. Page CB, Mostafa A, Saiao A, et al. Cardiovascular toxicity in levetiracetam overdose. Clinical Toxicology (Philadelphia). 2016;54(2):125–130.

Chapter 20
Hymenoptera Stings

Key Considerations

1. Hymenoptera stings cause approximately one to two deaths annually in Australia.

2. Their venom is a prevalent cause of allergic reactions and anaphylaxis, affecting around 3% of the population.

3. Anaphylaxis necessitates venom immunotherapy as a definitive treatment.

4. Though rare, extensive bee or wasp envenomation can result in multi-organ failure and death.

5. Ant stings are not commonly associated with mass envenomation.

Introduction

The Hymenoptera order consists of about 35,000 insect species, including bees, wasps, and ants from the families Apidae, Vespidae, and Formicidae. Clinical manifestations of their stings range from mild local irritation to severe allergic reactions, including anaphylaxis, which constitutes up to 35% of annual anaphylaxis cases. Approximately 3% of those stung experience anaphylaxis.

In Australia, Hymenoptera stings account for a comparable number of deaths as snake bites (averaging two per year) and lead to double the number of hospitalizations. Despite their impact, most bee and wasp species are solitary and seldom sting humans.

Bee Stings

The European honeybee (Apis mellifera) is the most common source of stings in Australia. Female honey bees sting once, leaving their stingers embedded. The venom contains melittin, which causes pain and local reactions.

Clinical Effects

The severity of symptoms depends on the bee species, prior exposure, and the individual's sensitivity:

Local Reactions:

Pain and irritation usually subside within 1–2 hours but may persist up to 48 hours.

Approximately 10% of cases involve large local reactions, peaking at 48 hours and lasting up to 10 days.

Anaphylaxis

Mediated by IgE antibodies, it typically occurs within 30 minutes of the sting, often within minutes.

Severe cases can manifest as prolonged or recurrent reactions lasting up to 24 hours.

This is the leading cause of death from Hymenoptera stings.

Other Effects

Serum sickness and mass envenomation are rare but significant complications.

Wasp Stings

Wasps are responsible for most single stings and Hymenoptera-related fatalities in the U.S. and Europe, though they cause fewer deaths than bees in Australia. Wasps are aggressive and capable of multiple stings. Swarming, triggered by chemical signals, can lead to life-threatening mass envenomation. Symptoms are similar to those caused by bee stings.

Mass Envenomation

Mass envenomation is rare and typically involves species like the African "killer bee" or European honeybee, often following the disturbance of a colony.

Diagnostic Threshold

> 50 bee stings (or 1–4 stings per kilogram in children).

> 20 wasp stings.

Clinical Features

Symptoms appear within 24 hours and may include:

Initial: Headache, weakness, lethargy, diarrhea, and vomiting.

Severe: Hemolysis, acute kidney and liver injury, rhabdomyolysis, ARDS, myocardial damage, DIC, and shock.

Mortality (~15%) is associated with more than 150 bee or 20 wasp stings. Rapid deaths are usually due to anaphylaxis.

Treatment

Single Stings: Remove stingers promptly (venom is injected within two minutes). Symptomatic relief includes cold compresses, analgesics, and antihistamines. Observation may be required for hypersensitivity.

Mass Envenomation: Remove all stingers rapidly. Admit patients for intensive supportive care, monitoring renal and hepatic function, electrolytes, and coagulation profiles.

Ant Stings

Ant stings cause pain and may induce systemic reactions. Medically significant species include:

1. Bull Ants (Myrmecia):

Found across southern Australia.

"Jack Jumper ants" are particularly notorious, causing local swelling and systemic allergic reactions in 3% of Australians, with 50% of cases being life-threatening.

2. Fire Ants (Solenopsis invicta):

Introduced to Australia in 2001, fire ants are highly aggressive and frequently swarm.

Stings can cause painful burning sensations and hypersensitivity reactions. Severe cases result in pustules, which should not be ruptured to prevent secondary infection.

3. Green Ants (Rhytidoponera metallica):

Native to Queensland, they can trigger severe allergic reactions.

Treatment

Manage allergic reactions using antihistamines or epinephrine for anaphylaxis.

Consider venom immunotherapy for patients with prior severe reactions.

Venom Immunotherapy

Venom-specific immunotherapy is the gold standard for individuals with a history of anaphylaxis caused by honeybees, paper wasps, European wasps, or Jack Jumper ants. While effective in preventing severe allergic reactions (80–90% success rate), it does not prevent localized symptoms.

References

1. Perez-Riverol A et al. (2015). Facing Hymenoptera venom allergy. Toxins.

2. Welton RE et al. (2017). Injury trends from envenoming in Australia. Intern Med J.

3. McGain F et al. (2000). Wasp sting mortality in Australia. Med J Aust.

4. Vetter RS et al. (1999). Mass envenomations by honeybees and wasps. West J Med.

5. Visscher PK et al. (1996). Removing bee stings. Lancet.

6. Brown SG et al. (2011). Causes of ant sting anaphylaxis in Australia. Med J Aust.

7. Queensland Government. (2016). Fire ants FAQ.

8. Solley GO et al. (2002). Anaphylaxis due to fire ants. Med J Aust.

Chapter 21
Toxidromes

Key Consideration

Anticholinergic (Antimuscarinic) Toxic Syndrome

Anticholinergic toxic syndrome (ACTS) arises from the inhibition of postsynaptic muscarinic receptors or the disruption of cholinergic transmission at these sites due to specific medications.

Serotonin Toxicity

Clonus, whether spontaneous, inducible, or ocular, is a hallmark sign of serotonin toxicity (ST), especially when a history of serotonergic agent ingestion is established. Key considerations include:

1. Interactions between selective serotonin reuptake inhibitors (SSRIs) and monoamine oxidase inhibitors (MAOIs) may result in life-threatening conditions necessitating immediate and aggressive intervention.

2. Dopamine agonists, such as bromocriptine (used for neuroleptic malignant syndrome), may exacerbate ST due to dual receptor activity on 5-HT and dopamine systems.

3. Fluoxetine can induce ST even weeks after discontinuation, particularly when combined with other serotonergic agents.

4. Clinical monitoring focuses on clonus and hyperreflexia for diagnostic confirmation.

Sympathomimetic Toxicity

The primary features of sympathomimetic toxidrome include agitation, repetitive behaviors, delirium, hypertension, tachycardia, hyperthermia, and pressured speech.

1. Tachycardia with diaphoresis and increased bowel sounds suggests adrenergic toxicity, whereas decreased sweating and urinary retention may indicate anticholinergic effects.

2. Patients on MAOIs or bupropion are at heightened risk for adrenergic toxicity, even at lower stimulant doses.

3. Management emphasizes supportive care, benzodiazepines, and vigilant monitoring for end-organ damage and hyperthermia.

Cholinergic Toxicity

Excessive stimulation of nicotinic and muscarinic receptors, or increased acetylcholine (ACh) transmission, underlies cholinergic toxicity.

1. Nicotinic effects often manifest as agitation, vomiting, seizures, arrhythmias, and paralysis leading to respiratory failure in severe cases.

2. Muscarinic agonists may cause symptoms such as bradycardia, excessive salivation, bronchospasm, and neurological signs like coma or convulsions.

3. Treatment is predominantly supportive, involving atropine and acetylcholinesterase (AChE) reactivators for significant organophosphate toxicity.

Anticholinergic Toxic Syndrome

Overview

ACTS occurs due to impaired cholinergic signaling at muscarinic receptors, often triggered by drug overdose, chronic medication use, or ingestion of certain plant alkaloids. The resultant cholinergic deficiency manifests in both central and peripheral symptoms.

Clinical Manifestations

Classic symptoms are summarized by the mnemonic "mad as a hatter, blind as a bat, red as a beet, hot as a hare, dry as a bone."

1. Peripheral Signs:

Dry mucous membranes

Tachycardia

Urinary retention

Reduced gastrointestinal motility

Blurred vision

Fever, stemming from diminished sweating, CNS dysregulation, or increased activity.

2. Central Symptoms:

Agitation

Confusion

Hallucinations

High-Risk Populations

Elderly individuals with reduced central cholinergic capacity.

Children with conditions like trisomy 21.

Patients with organic CNS disorders, such as dementia or Parkinson's disease.

Cases involving co-ingestion of agents with anticholinergic or multi-receptor actions, such as antipsychotics or antihistamines.

Common Culprit Agents

Medications: Antipsychotics (e.g., olanzapine, quetiapine), antihistamines (e.g., diphenhydramine), tricyclic antidepressants (e.g., amitriptyline).

Plants: Belladonna alkaloids and angel trumpet.

Prognostic Indicators

Outcomes are generally favorable in isolated ACTS cases, though co-ingestants may complicate recovery.

Fever correlates with larger ingestions and poorer outcomes.

Delirium severity can be graded using established scoring systems.

Management

Mild Cases

Benzodiazepines for agitation, with careful monitoring for respiratory depression or worsening delirium.

Moderate to Severe Cases

Physostigmine: Administered in titrated doses (0.5–1 mg IV) to reverse central effects like delirium, with close monitoring for complications such as seizures (risk ~1%).

Rivastigmine: Preferred for prolonged cases; slower onset but effective for moderate severity.

Peripheral Symptoms

Ileus or pseudo-obstruction may be treated with peripheral cholinesterase inhibitors like neostigmine.

Dose: 2.5 mg IV over 10–20 minutes.

Side effects include salivation, nausea, bradycardia, and bronchospasm.

Monitoring

Continuous cardiac monitoring is essential to detect potential arrhythmias or cardiotoxicity.

Comprehensive Analysis and Structured Overview of Toxicity Syndromes

1. Severity Scale for Central Nervous System Stimulation (CNS)

A structured grading system evaluates the severity of CNS stimulation, facilitating the appropriate clinical response based on observable findings:

Severity Score	Clinical Findings
0	Relaxed and cooperative behavior
1	Anxious, irritable and exhibiting tremors
2	Intermittent or mild confusion, hallucinations, moderate agitation and increased motor activity
3	Incoherent speech, significant agitation, marked motor hyperactive (often necessitating restraints)
4	Seizures or profound coma (unresponsive to pain or verbal stimuli)

This scale is adapted from clinical research on anticholinergic poisoning and has been validated in emergency settings (Burns et al., 2000).

2. Clinical Signs of Delirium in Anticholinergic Toxidrome

Anticholinergic toxidrome (ACTS) often manifests with CNS and peripheral symptoms. Diagnosis may require focused observation and testing:

Perceptual Abnormalities: Patients may misinterpret visual stimuli, such as picking at nonexistent objects or bed sheets.

Peripheral Signs: Symptoms such as salivation, bradycardia, diaphoresis, and lacrimation indicate excessive acetylcholinesterase (AChE) inhibition.

Treatment Considerations:

Avoid antipsychotics with anticholinergic properties (e.g., olanzapine, quetiapine).

Benzodiazepines and AChE inhibitors like physostigmine are effective options for managing profound delirium.

3. Serotonin Toxicity (Serotonin Syndrome)

Serotonin syndrome (ST) is characterized by excessive central serotonin activity, typically presenting within six hours of exposure to serotonergic agents. This condition is stratified by severity:

Clinical Triad:

1. Neuromuscular Excitation: Ocular/ankle clonus, myoclonus, hyperreflexia, rigidity.

2. Autonomic Excitation: Tachycardia, hyperthermia.

3. Altered Mental State: Agitation, confusion.

Mechanism: Overactivation of 5-HT2a receptors due to serotonergic agents, including selective serotonin reuptake inhibitors (SSRIs) and monoamine oxidase inhibitors (MAOIs).

Management:

Mild: Supportive care with or without activated charcoal.

Moderate: Sedation using midazolam or diazepam; cyproheptadine for serotonin antagonism.

Severe: Intubation, active cooling, and monitoring for complications (e.g., rhabdomyolysis, renal failure).

High-Risk Groups:

Patients on multiple serotonergic agents or CYP2D6 inhibitors.

Those genetically deficient in CYP2D6, increasing susceptibility to ST.

4. Sympathomimetic Toxicity

This condition arises from adrenergic receptor activation, often due to stimulant drugs like amphetamines or catecholamine release. Key features include:

Clinical Presentation:

Agitation, repetitive movements, pressured speech.

Tachycardia, hypertension, hyperthermia.

Neuropsychiatric symptoms such as paranoia or psychosis.

Complications:

End-organ damage, particularly with hyperthermia or rhabdomyolysis.

Management:

Benzodiazepines for sedation and muscle relaxation.

Supportive care to prevent hyperthermia and associated complications.

5. Prognostic Indicators

Across these syndromes, critical prognostic indicators guide treatment urgency:

CNS Stimulation: Escalation from mild agitation to seizures or coma requires immediate intervention.

Serotonin Syndrome: Hyperthermia >38.5°C and sustained clonus indicate severe toxicity.

Sympathomimetic Toxicity: Persistent symptoms beyond 24 hours or cardiac instability necessitate intensive care.

6. Monitoring and Discharge

Continuous observation is essential for moderate to severe cases, particularly for signs of cardiotoxicity, hyperthermia, or respiratory compromise:

Mild Cases: Can often be managed outpatient once asymptomatic.

Severe Cases: Require monitoring in intensive care settings until clinical stability is achieved.

Chapter 22
Chloroquine

Key Considerations

1. Chloroquine overdose is highly toxic and carries a significant mortality risk.

2. Cardiac toxicity can develop rapidly and may precede hospital arrival.

3. The primary treatment approach involves supportive care and the administration of adrenaline.

4. Early consultation with a toxicology expert is crucial for effective management.

5. Hospital admission and continuous cardiac monitoring are required for all cases of deliberate self-poisoning.

Introduction

Chloroquine is a medication commonly used for the treatment of malaria and certain autoimmune diseases. It has a chemical structure similar to quinidine, and another related compound, hydroxychloroquine, is often preferred in clinical settings due to its slightly lower toxicity. Both drugs exhibit similar toxicological profiles in cases of overdose, leading to similar treatment strategies. Chloroquine is predominantly used in regions where malaria is endemic, especially in low- and middle-income countries. However, in France, its use in self-poisoning has contributed significantly to understanding its life-threatening toxicity.

At the cellular level, chloroquine, like quinidine, stabilizes myocardial membranes by blocking voltage-gated ion channels for calcium (Ca^{2+}), sodium (Na^+), and potassium (K^+), which leads to negative inotropy, delayed conduction, and an elevated depolarization threshold within the heart muscle. These cardiac effects are the primary cause of its lethal potential in overdose cases.

Pharmacokinetics

Chloroquine is rapidly absorbed after oral ingestion, with peak blood levels typically reached within hours. The drug is widely distributed to extravascular tissues due to its large volume of distribution. Despite its long elimination half-life of 6 to 14 days, the most critical period for toxicity occurs within the first few hours post-ingestion. Blood concentrations of chloroquine correlate with clinical toxicity and mortality, though serum levels are not usually available quickly enough to influence real-time treatment decisions.

Clinical Manifestations

The most significant clinical concern following a chloroquine overdose is cardiac toxicity, which can manifest rapidly. The drug's toxic effects peak within hours, correlating with the highest blood concentrations. Key clinical features of toxicity include arrhythmias such as ventricular tachycardia and torsades de pointes, which can lead to cardiac arrest. Electrocardiographic changes, such as a QRS complex greater than 120 ms and prolonged QT intervals, are commonly observed. Hypotension, often due to myocardial depression, may be refractory to treatment.

Central nervous system (CNS) effects like seizures can occur, although they are less common than cardiac symptoms. A decreased level of consciousness may also be present, often exacerbated by coingestants like alcohol or sedative-hypnotic drugs. Additionally, severe hypokalemia can develop, likely caused by the redistribution of potassium across cellular membranes, rather than a deficiency in total body potassium.

Deaths can occur early due to cardiac arrest, with later fatalities typically resulting from refractory shock and complications associated with prolonged resuscitation efforts. A study in a high-income country with access to advanced critical care found an overall mortality rate just under 10%.

Management

Early risk assessment is crucial when managing chloroquine overdoses. Ingestions of greater than 5 grams are generally associated with a high likelihood of severe toxicity or death, but fatalities can also occur with lower doses. As such, all deliberate self-poisonings involving chloroquine should be treated as potentially fatal, with patients receiving high-priority triage (category 2 under the Australasian triage scale). Immediate cardiac monitoring is essential upon hospital arrival, and patients should be managed in a high-acuity setting with close observation.

Activated charcoal (50 grams) should be administered to conscious patients if they present within 1 hour of ingestion. If the patient presents later, charcoal may still be considered, especially if large quantities were ingested, although its efficacy diminishes with time. However, gastric lavage, a previously common method of decontamination, has become less favored in modern practice.

Blood tests should be performed early to assess potassium levels, as hypokalemia is a critical marker of toxicity. Continuous monitoring of vital signs and 12-lead ECGs is essential to track changes in cardiac function, such as QRS prolongation and QT interval lengthening. Early consultation with a toxicologist is recommended, as blood levels of chloroquine, though indicative of severity, are rarely available promptly enough for immediate clinical use.

Supportive Care

The cornerstone of chloroquine overdose management is supportive care. Early intubation and ventilation should be considered if the patient's condition deteriorates. The choice of sedative for intubation has been debated. For example, a study found that large doses of sodium thiopental used to facilitate intubation were associated with profound shock in some patients, leading to recommendations against its use. Ketamine, with its cardiac-stable properties, may be a better choice for intubation in these cases.

Diazepam has been historically suggested as beneficial in chloroquine poisoning, especially when used in conjunction with adrenaline, intubation, and mechanical ventilation for patients ingesting more than 5 grams of chloroquine. However, recent randomized controlled trials found no clear benefit of diazepam in improving survival rates or clinical outcomes compared to placebo.

Cardiovascular Management

Close monitoring of the patient's circulation is critical. Regular 12-lead ECGs should be conducted to detect any signs of toxicity, including prolonged QRS complexes and QT intervals. Hypotension is common, and a systolic blood pressure below 80 mm Hg is a significant risk factor for death. The primary cause of hypotension in these cases is likely toxin-induced cardiogenic shock due to chloroquine's negative inotropic effects. If hypotension develops, a crystalloid bolus (20 mL/kg) may be given to address potential hypovolemia, but the most appropriate intervention is the administration of adrenaline, which should be initiated early.

Adrenaline is the preferred inotrope, and can be administered via a peripheral venous access, provided the cannula is sufficiently large (18 gauge or greater) and the drug is diluted appropriately. A typical adrenaline infusion regimen begins with 0.25 µg/kg/min, with incremental adjustments as needed to achieve an adequate blood pressure.

Management of Hypokalemia

Hypokalemia, a common consequence of chloroquine toxicity, is thought to result from potassium redistribution, not a total body deficit. The use of adrenaline may worsen hypokalemia, and aggressive potassium replacement may risk rebound hyperkalemia once the acute toxicity resolves. Therefore, careful monitoring and titration of potassium levels are necessary in a critical care setting.

Additional Therapies

For patients who do not respond adequately to the initial management strategies, further interventions may be considered. Hypertonic sodium bicarbonate has been suggested to reverse the blockade of fast sodium channels in the heart and may be useful in patients with prolonged QRS intervals. Lipid emulsions have also been proposed as a treatment option, but evidence supporting their efficacy in chloroquine toxicity remains limited.

Conclusion

Management of chloroquine overdose requires rapid assessment and intervention. Early cardiac monitoring, supportive care, and the judicious use of inotropes like adrenaline are essential for improving outcomes. Although there is no specific antidote for chloroquine poisoning, advances in treatment protocols have improved survival rates, particularly when critical care resources are available. Consultation with a toxicologist should be sought early in the management of severe cases.

References

1. Riou B, Barriot P, Rimailho A, et al. Treatment of severe
chloroquine poisoning. N Engl J Med. 1988;318(1):1–6.

2. Michael TAD, Eivazzadeh S. The effects of acute -

quine poisoning with special reference to the heart. Am
Heart J. 1970;79(6):831–842.

3. Clemessy JL, Taboulet P, Hoffman JR, et al. Treatment
of acute chloroquine poisoning: a 5-year experience. Crit
Care Med. 1996;24(7):1189–1195.

4. Bagate F, Radu C, Mekontso Dessap A, de Prost N. Early
extracorporeal membrane oxygenation for -
lar failure in a patient with massive chloroquine poisoning. Am J Emerg Med. 2017;35(2):380.e3–380.e4.

5. Clemessy JL, Borron SW, Baud FJ, et al. Hypokalemia related to acute chloroquine ingestion. Lancet.
1995;346(8979):877–880.

6. Clemessy JL, Angel G, Borron SW, et al. Therapeutic trial of diazepam versus placebo in acute chloroquine intoxications of moderate gravity. Intensive Care Med. 1996;22(12). 1400–1045.

7. Marquardt K, Albertson TE. Treatment of -quine overdose. Am J Emerg Med. 2001;19(5):420–424.

8. Höjer J, Jacobsen D, Neuvonen PJ, Rosenberg PH. Lipid rescue—efficacy and safety still unproven. Basic Clin Pharmacol Toxicol. 2016;119(4):345–348.

9. Sin JH, Tom A, Toyoda A, et al. High-dose intravenous lipid emulsion affecting successful initiation of continuous venovenous hemofiltration and extractor-

membrane oxygenation. Clin Toxicol (Phila). 2017;56(2):149–150.

Chapter 23
Opioids

Key Congratulations

1. Opioid Toxicity: Opioid toxicity typically presents with respiratory depression, altered consciousness, and pinpoint pupils (miosis).

2. Treatment Approach: The primary treatment for opioid toxicity involves naloxone administration and supportive care.

3. Other Toxic Effects: Certain opioids may induce additional toxic effects. For instance, tramadol can lead to seizures, methadone may cause QT interval prolongation, and dextropropoxyphene can result in QRS complex widening.

4. Pediatric Exposure: Children are particularly vulnerable to opioid toxicity, and overdose can lead to significant morbidity and mortality.

Introduction

Opioids are a broad class of substances, with morphine being the prototypical example. These include both prescription and illicit drugs that are widely used to manage acute and chronic pain. Opioids can be classified into short-acting and long-acting formulations, and they are administered through various routes, such as oral, intravenous, subcutaneous, buccal, inhaled, and transcutaneous. Opioids are a leading cause of drug-related deaths in Australia. Since 2007, the rate of accidental opioid deaths among Australians aged 35 to 44 has more than doubled, with a significant majority of these deaths attributed to prescription opioids, rather than heroin. The primary cause of death in opioid overdose cases is respiratory depression, which leads to hypoxia. Notably, deaths can occur many hours after opioid ingestion, particularly with long-acting formulations, if patients are not carefully monitored.

Additionally, various opioids can produce other toxic effects (see Table 25.23.1).

Pharmacology

Opioid drugs primarily exert their effects in the central and peripheral nervous systems. They act as agonists on different types of opioid receptors, with the mu opioid receptor being primarily responsible for their therapeutic and toxic effects. These receptors are distributed widely, including in the gastrointestinal tract, cardiovascular, and immune systems. Some opioids also affect non-opioid receptors, which can contribute to additional toxic effects in overdose situations. For example, tramadol inhibits both serotonin and norepinephrine reuptake, while methadone blocks the hERG potassium channel.

Pharmacokinetics among opioids vary considerably. For example, the bioavailability of buprenorphine is low at 10% (via oral route), while oxycodone has a high bioavailability of

70% (see Table 25.23.1). The onset of toxicity is dependent on the administration route, with intravenous administration resulting in rapid absorption (within minutes), intramuscular injections taking about an hour, and oral ingestion reaching peak concentrations within two hours. Opioids are predominantly metabolized in the liver by the cytochrome P450 system and conjugating enzymes, leading to both active and inactive metabolites. The duration of action varies significantly depending on the opioid formulation. Long-acting opioids, such as oral controlled-release morphine and oxycodone, or transdermal fentanyl, may have a prolonged absorption and extended toxicity.

Clinical Effects

The key clinical signs of opioid toxicity include miosis, central nervous system depression (ranging from drowsiness to coma), and respiratory depression. Common side effects also include nausea and vomiting. It is important to note that some opioids have additional, non-opioid-specific toxic effects. For example, tramadol in overdose frequently causes seizures, while methadone can lead to QT interval prolongation and dextropropoxyphene can block sodium channels, potentially causing cardiac arrhythmias.

Opioid toxicity can also lead to various complications due to their sedative and respiratory depressive effects. These include aspiration, non-cardiogenic pulmonary edema, rhabdomyolysis (due to prolonged immobility), compartment syndrome, acute renal injury, and hypoxic brain damage.

Management

The treatment of opioid toxicity involves supportive care and the administration of naloxone, an opioid antagonist. Ensuring adequate airway management and respiratory support is essential. The patient's respiratory rate should be carefully monitored, as individuals who are opioid-dependent may appear responsive but still suffer from respiratory depression that necessitates intervention.

Naloxone Administration

Naloxone is an opioid receptor antagonist that can be administered intravenously, intramuscularly, or intranasally. The dose is typically titrated based on the patient's respiratory rate, oxygen saturation, and level of consciousness. Naloxone usually produces a rapid response to opioid toxicity, but if hypoxic brain injury, co-ingestion, or other complications are present, response may be slower. The elimination half-life of naloxone is 60-90 minutes, which may be shorter than the half-life of the opioids involved. This means that repeated doses or a naloxone infusion may be required. In opioid-dependent individuals, naloxone administration can precipitate withdrawal, which may cause agitation, so smaller doses should be used to avoid abrupt opioid reversal.

For short-acting opioids, a single dose of naloxone is often sufficient. However, for long-acting opioids (e.g., methadone) or slow-release formulations, an infusion may be necessary to maintain clinical effect, which should be titrated based on the patient's respiratory rate and level of consciousness.

Opioids in Children

Children are at an increased risk for opioid toxicity due to pharmacokinetic differences from adults, such as variations in drug absorption, distribution, and metabolism. Accidental exposures to opioids, often from medications prescribed to adults, are a leading cause of pediatric toxicity. In fact, opioid exposures in children typically occur in the home setting. Notably, the number of pediatric overdoses is proportionate to the number of opioid prescriptions and their associated dosages. Accidental opioid ingestion in children can result in severe and prolonged toxicity, highlighting the critical importance of proper medication safety education.

Specific Opioid Agents

Buprenorphine

Buprenorphine is a partial opioid agonist with a high affinity for the mu receptor and a long duration of action. It has a "ceiling effect," meaning that increasing doses do not produce additional respiratory depression beyond a certain point. This makes it potentially safer in comparison to other opioids. However, co-ingestion with sedative agents or high doses can still cause significant toxicity, and larger amounts of naloxone may be needed to reverse its effects. Buprenorphine exposure in children has been linked to severe toxicity, even from minimal exposure, such as a single lick of a tablet.

Fentanyl

Fentanyl is an extremely potent synthetic opioid, 100 times stronger than morphine, and is used for both acute and chronic pain management. It is typically administered parenterally, via transmucosal routes, or transdermally. Due to its potency, even small amounts can lead to significant toxicity. Fentanyl has low oral bioavailability, but large doses or exposure through mucosal surfaces can result in severe toxicity. Fentanyl's half-life is approximately 3 hours, but its effects are typically much shorter, due to redistribution from the plasma. Fentanyl patches can contain large quantities of the drug, and misuse, such as injecting or swallowing the contents of a patch, can lead to prolonged toxicity and death.

Methadone

Methadone is a long-acting synthetic opioid with complex pharmacokinetics, which can vary widely between individuals. It is primarily used in opioid substitution therapy and can take several days to stabilize a patient on an appropriate dose. Methadone is known to prolong the QT interval, which can increase the risk of torsades de pointes, especially at higher doses or when combined with other QT-prolonging medications. Methadone metabolism can be affected by other drugs, leading to changes in plasma concentration, either increasing the risk of overdose or precipitating withdrawal symptoms.

Tramadol

Tramadol is a synthetic opioid with dual mechanisms of action: weak opioid receptor agonism and inhibition of serotonin and norepinephrine reuptake. In overdose, tramadol can lead to seizures and serotonin toxicity, particularly if combined with other serotonergic medications. Its metabolism produces an active metabolite, O-desmethyltramadol, which contributes to its analgesic effects.

Conclusion

Opioid toxicity is a frequently encountered condition in toxicology, marked by symptoms such as respiratory depression, reduced consciousness, and pinpoint pupils. The primary approach to managing opioid toxicity involves supportive care and the administration of naloxone. Additionally, it is essential to recognize and address the potential non-opioid effects associated with opioid use.

Chapter 24
Oral Anticoagulants

Key Considerations

1. Overdose Effects: All oral anticoagulants increase the International Normalized Ratio (INR) when overdosed, although the relationship may not be strictly dose-dependent.

2. Activated Charcoal: Activated charcoal can reduce absorption if apixaban is ingested, and it is likely effective for warfarin, dabigatran, and rivaroxaban as well.

3. Warfarin Management: Clear guidelines exist for managing warfarin overdose, and these should be adhered to consistently.

4. Reversal Agents: Prothrombinex-VF can reverse the effects of warfarin and rivaroxaban,

but it is not effective for dabigatran and may only partially reverse apixaban toxicity.

5. Idarucizumab: This agent is the preferred treatment for major bleeding caused by dabigatran.

6. Rivaroxaban Toxicity: Data on acute rivaroxaban overdose suggest that it is often less harmful due to its limited absorption rate.

Introduction

The primary oral anticoagulants currently available are warfarin, dabigatran, apixaban, and rivaroxaban. These include both direct thrombin inhibitors (dabigatran) and factor Xa inhibitors (apixaban and rivaroxaban), offering advantages like fixed dosing regimens and no requirement for routine coagulation monitoring. Compared to warfarin, which requires careful monitoring and dose adjustments, newer oral anticoagulants

(NOACs) or direct oral anticoagulants (DOACs) have been studied for their efficacy in preventing thromboembolic events. For patients with atrial fibrillation, apixaban has shown a slightly better therapeutic effect than warfarin in preventing thromboembolic events, although it does not significantly reduce stroke risk more effectively. Apixaban also demonstrates a significantly lower risk of major bleeding compared to warfarin, dabigatran, and rivaroxaban.

Pharmacology

Warfarin: Warfarin works by inhibiting the synthesis of vitamin K-dependent clotting factors. It is typically used for preventing venous thromboembolism (VTE), managing prosthetic heart valves, and preventing strokes in patients with atrial fibrillation (AF). It has a long half-life of 36-48 hours, with effects taking 3-5 days to manifest. Warfarin is primarily eliminated through the liver.

Dabigatran: Dabigatran directly inhibits thrombin, the enzyme responsible for fibrin production and platelet aggregation. It is used for VTE prevention after major surgeries like total hip replacement (THR) or total knee replacement (TKR), as well as for stroke prevention in high-risk AF patients. Dabigatran's half-life is around 12-14 hours, with most of its elimination through the kidneys (80%).

Apixaban: Apixaban inhibits factor Xa, a key component in the coagulation cascade. Like dabigatran, it is used for preventing VTE following major surgeries and managing AF in high-risk patients. It has a half-life of 8-15 hours, with a significant portion of its elimination occurring through the liver (75%) and kidneys (25%).

Rivaroxaban: Similar to apixaban, rivaroxaban inhibits factor Xa and is used for VTE prevention and AF management. Its half-life is between 7-13 hours, with 75% eliminated through the kidneys and 25% via the liver.

Mechanism of Action

All the oral anticoagulants interfere with the final pathway of coagulation, which includes the activation of factor X and the formation of a stable fibrin clot. Warfarin specifically affects factors VII and IX of the intrinsic pathway, further inhibiting the clotting process.

Clinical Features:

When used therapeutically, NOACs do not seem to significantly increase the risk of bleeding compared to warfarin. However, there are limited cases of overdose and poisoning with these drugs. For instance, dabigatran overdose cases have been reported, with doses ranging from 1,500 mg to 18,750 mg (the usual daily dose is 300 mg). In some cases, the INR was greater than 6.5, but only a few cases involved significant bleeding. In cases of rivaroxaban poisoning, there were no major bleeding events even with elevated INR levels. Apixaban overdose, with doses such as 200 and 300 mg, resulted in only minor bleeding and moderate INR elevation.

Clinical Investigation

In cases of oral anticoagulant overdose, the INR is typically elevated, correlating with the plasma concentration of the anticoagulant. Drug levels are not routinely tested as part of standard treatment, as they do not significantly influence management. For warfarin over-anticoagulation, an INR greater than 10 (even without bleeding) is considered an indicator for the administration of a prothrombin complex concentrate (PCC). Similar guidelines could potentially be applied to NOAC overdoses.

Treatment

The initial steps in treating anticoagulant overdose focus on stabilizing the patient, including managing active bleeding and performing fluid resuscitation if necessary. If the patient is not at risk of airway compromise, gastrointestinal decontamination with activated charcoal may be considered, especially within 1-2 hours of ingestion. Activated charcoal has been shown to reduce absorption in cases of apixaban overdose and is likely effective for other NOACs as well.

For warfarin, the use of vitamin K and prothrombin complex concentrate is well established in cases of major bleeding or life-threatening over-anticoagulation. While NOACs lack universally accepted guidelines, similar strategies using prothrombin complex concentrates (like Prothrombinex-VF) have been proposed for the reversal of their anticoagulant effects in the event of significant bleeding or life-threatening situations. Specific agents such as idarucizumab are the treatment of choice for reversing dabigatran toxicity. The use of PCC is under investigation for other NOACs, but there is no definitive consensus on the best approach yet.

In conclusion, while oral anticoagulants like warfarin and newer agents such as dabigatran, apixaban, and rivaroxaban offer therapeutic benefits, managing overdose requires careful consideration. Understanding the pharmacokinetics and pharmacodynamics of these agents, along with established guidelines for their reversal, is crucial for safe and effective patient management.

References

1. Australian Medicines Handbook 2018 [Internet]. Australian Medicines Handbook Pty Ltd.; 2018. Available from: https://amhonline.amh.net.au/. Accessed on April 28, 2018.

2. Holzmacher JL, Sarani B. Indications and techniques for anticoagulation reversal. Surg Clin North Am. 2017;97(6):1291–1305.

3. Proietti M, Romanazzi I, Romiti GF, et al. Apixaban usage for stroke prevention in atrial fibrillation: a systematic review and meta-analysis. Stroke. 2018;49(1):98–106.

4. Bundhun PK, Soogund MXS, Teeluck AR, et al. Bleeding risks associated with rivaroxaban and dabigatran in atrial fibrillation treatment: a systematic review and meta-analysis. BMC Cardiovasc Disord. 2017;17:9.

5. Stevenson JW, Minns AB, Smollin C, et al. Observational case series on dabigatran and rivaroxaban exposures reported to poison control centers. Am J Emerg Med. 2014;32(9):1077–1084.

6. Vlad I, Armstrong J, Ridgley J, Pascu O. Deliberate overdose of dabigatran: two case reports and laboratory monitoring recommendations. Clin Toxicol (Phila). 2016;54(3):286–289.

7. Peetermans M, Pollack Jr C, Reilly P, et al. Idarucizumab in dabigatran overdose management. Clin Toxicol (Phila). 2016;54(8):644–646.

8. Spiller HA, Mowry JB, Aleguas Jr A, et al. Observational study on factor Xa inhibitors rivaroxaban and apixaban reported to poison centers. Ann Emerg Med. 2016;67(2):189–195.

9. Kubitza D, Becka M, Roth A, Mueck W. Dose-escalation study on pharmacokinetics and pharmacodynamics of rivaroxaban in healthy elderly subjects. Curr Med Res Opin. 2008;24:2757–2765.

10. Barton J, Wong A, Graudins A. Anti-Xa activity in apixaban overdose: a case report. Clin Toxicol (Phila). 2016;54(9):871–873.

11. Leikin SM, Patel H, Welker KL, et al. No significant bleeding after acute apixaban overdose. Am J Emerg Med. 2017;35(5):801.e5–e6.

12. Tran HA, Chunilal SD, Harper PL, et al. Update on consensus guidelines for warfarin reversal. Med J Aust. 2013;198(4):198–199.

13. Therapeutic Guidelines Limited 2018 [Internet]. Therapeutic Guidelines Limited; 2018. Available from: https://tgldcdp.tg.org.au.acs.hcn.com.au/viewTopic?topicfile=anticoagulant-therapy&sectionId=cvg7-c31-s15-cvg7-c31-s15-5. Accessed on April 28, 2018.

14. Behring C. Prothrombinex®-VF Data Sheet 2018; 2018. Available from: http://www.cslbehring.com.au/.

15. Pisters R, Lane DA, Nieuwlaat R, de Vos CB, Crijns HJ, Lip GY. HAS-BLED score: A user-friendly tool to assess 1-year risk of major bleeding in atrial fibrillation. Chest. 2010;138(5):1093–1100.

16. Mangram A, Oguntodu OF, Dzandu JK, et al. Efficacy, safety, and cost-effectiveness comparison between 3-factor and 4-factor prothrombin complexes concentrated among trauma patients on oral anticoagulants. J Crit Care. 2016;33:252–256.

17. Martin DT, Barton CA, Dodgion C, Schreiber M. Emergent reversal of vitamin K antagonists: addressing all factors. Am J Surg. 2016;211(5):919–925.

18. Eerenberg ES, Kamphuisen PW, Sijpkens MK, et al. Reversal of rivaroxaban and dabigatran with prothrombin complex concentrate: a randomized, placebo-controlled, crossover study in healthy subjects. Circulation. 2011;124(14):1573–1579.

19. Awad NI, Brunetti L, Juurlink DN. Enhanced elimination of dabigatran via extracorporeal methods. J Med Toxicol. 2015;11(1):85–95.

20. Pollack Jr CV, Reilly PA, van Ryn J, et al. Idarucizumab for dabigatran reversal: full cohort analysis. N Engl J Med. 2017;377(5):431–441.

21. Tummala R, Kavtaradze A, Gupta A, Ghosh RK. Specific antidotes for direct oral anticoagulants: a comprehensive review of clinical trial data. Int J Cardiol. 2016;214:292–298.

Glossary

Activated Charcoal: A treatment used to reduce absorption of certain toxins in the gastrointestinal tract by adsorption, often administered in cases of drug overdoses.

Anticholinergic Toxic Syndrome (ACTS): A condition caused by the inhibition of muscarinic receptors, leading to symptoms such as dry skin, dilated pupils, and confusion.

Anticoagulants: Medications used to prevent blood clot formation; toxicity can result in increased bleeding risk, managed with specific reversal agents like Prothrombinex-VF or idarucizumab.

Chloroquine Toxicity: Overdose of chloroquine, a drug primarily used for malaria, associated with rapid-onset cardiac toxicity and a high risk of fatality.

Clonus: Repeated, involuntary muscle contractions, a key diagnostic feature of serotonin toxicity.

Envenomation: The injection of venom through a bite or sting, which can cause systemic reactions ranging from mild pain to multi-organ failure or anaphylaxis.

Glyphosate: A widely used herbicide whose surfactant co-formulants are implicated in cases of severe poisoning.

Hyperreflexia: An exaggerated reflex response, often observed in serotonin toxicity and indicative of central nervous system involvement.

International Normalized Ratio (INR): A measure of blood clotting used to monitor anticoagulant therapy; elevated levels indicate overdose or risk of bleeding.

Naloxone: An opioid antagonist used to reverse life-threatening respiratory depression caused by opioid overdose.

Paraquat: A highly toxic herbicide that causes fatal multi-organ failure or pulmonary fibrosis upon ingestion, with no effective antidote available.

Prothrombinex-VF: A clotting factor concentrate used to reverse the effects of anticoagulants like warfarin and rivaroxaban.

Serotonin Toxicity (ST): A potentially fatal condition caused by excessive serotonergic activity, commonly resulting from drug interactions between SSRIs and MAOIs.

Toxidrome: A clinical syndrome characterized by a specific set of signs and symptoms that suggest poisoning by a particular class of toxic substances.

Venom Immunotherapy (VIT): A treatment used to desensitize individuals with a history of anaphylaxis from Hymenoptera stings.

Wernicke Encephalopathy (WE): A neurological disorder resulting from thiamine deficiency, frequently seen in chronic alcohol abuse, requiring urgent thiamine supplementation.

www.ingramcontent.com/pod-product-compliance
Lightning Source LLC
Chambersburg PA
CBHW071017240526
45469CB00006BD/1952